T0200725

The Long Struggle Against Malaria in Tropical Africa

This book is the first history of malaria control efforts in tropical Africa. It is a contribution to the emerging subdiscipline of the historical epidemiology of contemporary disease challenges.

The Long Struggle Against Malaria in Tropical Africa investigates the changing entomological, parasitological, and medical understandings of vectors, parasites, and malarial disease that have shaped the programs of malaria control and altered the transmission of malarial infections. It examines the history of malaria control and eradication in the contexts of racial thought, population movements, demographic growth, economic change, urbanization, warfare, and politics. It will be useful for students of medicine and public health, for those who are involved with malaria research studies, and for those who work on the contemporary malaria control and elimination campaigns in tropical Africa.

James L. A. Webb, Jr., is professor of history at Colby College, where he teaches African health history and global health history. He is the recipient of a National Institutes of Health/National Library of Medicine Grant for Scholarly Writing in Biomedicine and Health. His books include *Global Health in Africa: Historical Perspectives on Disease Control* (2013), edited with T. Giles-Vernick, and *Humanity's Burden: A Global History of Malaria* (2009). His articles have appeared in *The Lancet, Journal of the History of Medicine and Allied Sciences, Journal of African History, Journal of World History,* and *Environmental History.*

The Long Struggle Against Malaria in Tropical Africa

JAMES L. A. WEBB, JR.
Colby College

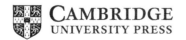
CAMBRIDGE
UNIVERSITY PRESS

CAMBRIDGE
UNIVERSITY PRESS

32 Avenue of the Americas, New York, NY 10013–2473, USA

Cambridge University Press is part of the University of Cambridge.

It furthers the University's mission by disseminating knowledge in the pursuit of education, learning, and research at the highest international levels of excellence.

www.cambridge.org
Information on this title: www.cambridge.org/9781107052574

First published 2014

Printed in the United States of America

A catalog record for this publication is available from the British Library.

Library of Congress Cataloging in Publication Data
Webb, James L. A., Jr., 1952– author.
The long struggle against malaria in tropical Africa / James L.A. Webb Jr.
p. ; cm.
Includes bibliographical references and index.
ISBN 978-1-107-05257-4 (hardback)
I. Title.
[DNLM: 1. Malaria – history – Africa South of the Sahara. 2. Malaria – prevention & control – Africa South of the Sahara. 3. Disease Eradication – history – Africa South of the Sahara. 4. History, 20th Century – Africa South of the Sahara. 5. History, 21st Century – Africa South of the Sahara. 6. Mosquito Control – history – Africa South of the Sahara. WC 765]
RA644.M2
614.5'320967–dc23   2013048022

ISBN 978-1-107-05257-4 Hardback

In memory of
Philip D. Curtin (1922–2009)
A pioneer in historical epidemiology

Contents

Maps

Photographs

Illustration and Table

x

Preface

The Long Struggle Against Malaria in Tropical Africa is about the history of efforts to control malaria in tropical Africa from the beginnings of modern scientific knowledge about the disease in the late nineteenth century to the present. It is intended as a contribution to the emerging subdiscipline of the historical epidemiology of contemporary disease challenges. It investigates the changing medical understandings of the disease and explores the changing entomological and parasitological understandings that have shaped the programs of malaria control and altered the transmission of malaria. It examines the history of malaria control in the contexts of racial thought, population movements, demographic growth, economic change, urbanization, warfare, and politics. The goal is to blend disciplinary approaches and knowledge in a historical epidemiology that will be useful for students of medicine and public health, for those who are involved with malaria research studies, and for those who work on the contemporary malaria control and elimination campaigns in tropical Africa.

The book reveals a long history of well-intentioned malaria interventions that have been allowed to lapse. When a high degree of control over malaria transmission has been lost, epidemic malaria has afflicted age cohorts that had previously been protected by virtue of their acquired immunities. In this sense, the aftermaths of the lapsed projects cannot be accurately characterized as the re-establishment of a prior pattern of transmission or a state of equilibrium. This historical perspective on malaria control has been developed in part through the consultation of archival materials that are not available through PubMed and thus are largely unknown to the biomedical community.

The Long Struggle Against Malaria in Tropical Africa highlights the central issue of acquired immunity. Early in the twentieth century, European-trained physicians recognized a principal epidemiological difference between the response of nonimmune Europeans and partially immune Africans to malarial infection. The nature, role, and duration of the immunological response after initial infection were of critical importance in shaping malaria interventions. In the interwar period, European assumptions about the significance of acquired immunity helped to determine whether Africans should receive chemical therapies and, if so, the dosage regimens that were appropriate.

The issue of acquired immunity re-emerged in the immediate aftermath of the Second World War, when a highly successful malaria control effort in Freetown, Sierra Leone, lapsed and malaria resurged. It was central to the debates over whether to attempt the eradication of malaria in rural Africa during the build-up to the Global Malaria Eradication Program (GMEP) of the World Health Organization (WHO). It re-emerged again, following the closure of the WHO malaria eradication pilot projects, when resurgent malaria struck some of the populations that had been protected from infection during the life of the pilot projects. It looms as an issue in the context of contemporary campaigns to control or eliminate malaria as commitments in some quarters to sustaining the gains from malaria interventions have waned.

The Long Struggle Against Malaria in Tropical Africa is organized chronologically. "An Introduction to African Malaria" presents some deep historical background on the emergence of African malaria infections and genetic mutations to malarial pressure and provides historical context for understanding the role of acquired immunity in tropical Africa. The first two chapters are focused on the first half of the twentieth century. "European Vulnerability" discusses the arrival of Europeans in tropical Africa and examines the efforts that Europeans took to protect themselves from malaria, including the establishment of separate residential neighborhoods in coastal towns. It discusses the early European projects in mosquito control and the European efforts to improve the health of Africans who worked directly for Europeans in mining enclaves or who lived in urban environments. "African Immunity" introduces African efforts at mosquito control and African antimalarials and explores European knowledge and attitudes toward African malarial infections and treatment in rural environments, including European-owned farms and plantations. The discovery of African adult acquired immunity and African childhood vulnerability raised fundamental questions for European colonial medical officers about how to address the "African" malaria problem.

The third chapter, "An Aborted Campaign for Eradication," examines tropical Africa's malaria control and eradication pilot projects during the era of the global malaria eradication campaign (1950–1965) that was overseen by the WHO. The projects, based on the use of synthetic insecticides for indoor residual house-spraying, dramatically reduced malaria in endemic zones but could not sustain the interruption of transmission because mosquito resistance to the insecticides emerged and the projects did not have the full support of African populations in the project zones.

The fourth chapter, "Positive Turbulence," investigates the unexpected malaria dynamics of the early era of independence (1965–1980) in much of former British and French colonial Africa. Independent African governments did not embrace the WHO's vision of pre-eradication malaria programs, preferring to allocate scarce resources to other medical problems, yet deaths from malaria declined. This was in good measure owing to the widespread availability of the inexpensive antimalarial drug chloroquine and to the rapid urbanization of tropical Africa.

The fifth chapter, "Silent Resurgence," explores the last two decades of the twentieth century, when the broad use of chemical therapies selected for drug-resistant malaria parasites and signaled the end of an era. The dramatic decline of the efficacy of chloroquine, in particular, caused malaria death rates in children to climb precipitously. This chapter also examines the rise of synergistic infections with human immunodeficiency virus (HIV) and tuberculosis in the context of the weakening public health infrastructure seen throughout much of Africa.

The sixth chapter, "The Campaign for Elimination," discusses the twenty-first-century commitment to fighting malaria in Africa, one that depends on the continued efficacy of a new class of antimalarial drugs based on the alkaloid artemisinin and on the widespread distribution of insecticide-treated bed nets. It examines the new hopes for eventual eradication that are based on a new paradigm of "elimination." It explores contemporary control efforts in light of the ongoing processes of urbanization and the limitations posed by ongoing civil conflict in Africa.

A final reflection, "Perspectives," compares the difficulties that have been encountered in past malaria control and eradication interventions with those in the current campaigns. It emphasizes the need for those involved in planning contemporary control and eradication programs to design and implement safeguards against the resurgence of malaria.

Acknowledgments

The Long Struggle Against Malaria in Tropical Africa is based in part on research conducted in the Archives de l'Ecole du Pharo at the Institut de Médicine Tropicale du Service de Santé des Armées in Marseille, the Ross Archives of the London School of Hygiene and Tropical Medicine, the National Archives of the United Kingdom in Kew, the Rhodes House Library at the University of Oxford, the Malaria Room of the Wellcome Unit for the History of Medicine at the University of Oxford, the Contemporary Medical Archives Center of the Wellcome Library in London, and the Parasitological Archives of the World Health Organization in Geneva. I am deeply grateful to the archivists and staff of these institutions. I would like to thank in particular Marie Villemin Partow, an archivist at the World Health Organization, who was unstinting in her efforts to ensure that I had access to the classified and unclassified malaria materials that were relevant for this project.

This book developed from an earlier research project on the global history of malaria. During an initial research stint at the Wellcome Unit for the History of Medicine at Oxford, I had the good fortune to be introduced to research materials that had been gathered by a team of eminent scholars who had initiated and then abandoned a project on the history of malaria in East Africa. At the Wellcome Unit, I had a first inkling that it might be possible to write a broad historical epidemiology of African malaria. I am grateful to Mark Harrison, the Director of the Wellcome Unit, for facilitating my visits in Oxford.

The archival research for this book was funded, in part, by financial assistance from Social Science Division Grants from Colby College over the course of several years. I appreciate the confidence of the Grants

Committee and the support of Ed Yeterian and Lori Kletzer, the successive Deans of Faculty. The Wellcome Trust provided a grant that allowed me to defray my expenses during a semester of research in London, Oxford, and Geneva. I would like to express my appreciation to Geoff Targett of the London School of Hygiene and Tropical Medicine, who suggested that I approach the Wellcome Trust, and to Tony Woods at the Wellcome Trust, who facilitated the grant.

I am grateful for a grant for Scholarly Writing in Biomedicine and Health from the National Library of Medicine of the National Institutes of Health. It purchased two semesters of release from teaching that provided the time to write this book.[1]

I have presented some of the arguments in this book at symposia and invited lectures. I would like to thank my hosts for their invitations to visit their institutions and for many illuminating formal and informal sessions: Sharon Abramowitz at the University of Florida, Liliana Andonova at the Graduate Institute of International and Development Studies (Geneva), Lindsay Braun and Melissa Graboyes at the University of Oregon, John Brooke at Ohio State University, Peter Brown and Mari Webel at the Institute for Developing Nations at Emory University, Clifton Crais at Emory University, Elizabeth Eames and Leslie Hill at Bates College, Myron Echenberg at McGill University, Elfatih Eltahir at the Massachusetts Institute of Technology, Tamara Giles-Vernick and Ken Vernick at the Institut Pasteur (Paris), David Gordon at Bowdoin College, Mark Harrison at the University of Oxford, Marcelo Jacobs-Lorena at the Johns Hopkins Bloomberg School of Public Health, Emmanuel Kreike at Princeton University, Alan Magill at the Bill and Melinda Gates Foundation, Anouar Majid at the University of New England, Jim McCann at Boston University, Sheryl McCurdy at the University of Texas School of Public Health in Houston, Rod McIntosh at Yale University, Amanda Kay McVety at Miami University of Ohio, Frank Richards and Amy Patterson at The Carter Center, Clive Shiff and Nina Martin at the Johns Hopkins Malaria Research Institute, Frank Snowden at Yale University, Kerry Ward at Rice University, Bob Wirtz at the Centers for Disease Control, Tim Ziemer at the President's Malaria

[1] Funding for this project was made possible by grant 1G13LM10888–02 from the National Library of Medicine, NIH, DHHS. The views expressed in any written publication or other media do not necessarily reflect the official policies of the Department of Health and Human Services; nor does mention by trade names, commercial practices, or organizations imply endorsement by the United States.

Initiative/USAID, and Patrick Zylberman at the Ecoles des Hautes Etudes en Santé Publique (Paris).

An earlier and abbreviated version of Chapter 3, presented at a Yale symposium, appeared as "Malaria Control and Eradication Projects in Tropical Africa, 1945–1965," in Rick Bucala and Frank Snowden (eds.), *The Global Challenge of Malaria: Past Lessons and Future Prospects* (New York: World Scientific Publishing, 2014).

Over years of research, I have greatly benefited from conversations with malaria specialists who advance the work of governments, non-governmental organizations, international agencies, and university research centers. I have also been deeply enriched by my conversations with historians of medicine, Africanist historians, environmental historians, ecologists, entomologists, parasitologists, physicians, and public health specialists. I am appreciative of countless helpful conversations and challenges to ideas and assumptions. In addition to the scholars mentioned above, I would like to thank Jean-Paul Bado, Sanjoy Bhattacharya, David Bradley, Kent Campbell, Hal Cook, Dana Dalrymple, Monica Green, Rich Hoffmann, Al Howard, Margaret Humphreys, Bill Jobin, Tony Kiszewski, Christian Lengeler, Socrates Litsios, Michael Macdonald, Greg Maddox, Stuart McCook, Louis Molineaux, Pepe Nájera, Randy Packard, Rich Pollack, Andrew Read, Aafje Rietveld, Alan Schapira, and Geoff Targett for their willingness to discuss a wide variety of technical and historical issues. I have learned from them all.

I would like to thank Bill Jobin for inviting me to participate in the quarterly meetings of a multidisciplinary working group on African malaria and Jim McCann for inviting me to participate in the deliberations of the team of Rockefeller Foundation–funded researchers who investigated the impact of the adoption of hybrid maize in Ethiopia. The exchanges among researchers from a broad range of disciplinary backgrounds were enriching.

Two anonymous reviewers for Cambridge University Press made helpful suggestions to improve the manuscript. I offer my special thanks to Tamara Giles-Vernick, Michael Macdonald, Randy Packard, and Rich Pollack who graciously provided detailed commentary on a draft of the entire book manuscript.

My devoted wife, Alison Jones Webb, read the final draft with close attention to passages in which I could express my ideas more clearly and to transitions between ideas that I could address more smoothly. Her companionship and love have been vital in bringing this research to publication.

Glossary

Anophelines: Mosquitoes of the genus *Anopheles*. Some species in this genus are capable of hosting and transmitting the malaria parasites to human beings.

Anthrophily: The propensity of the female of mosquito species to prefer a blood meal from *Homo sapiens sapiens* (human beings) to that from another animal species. These propensities vary among anopheline species and are an important determinant of vector capacity to transmit malaria.

Bionomics: The study of ecological variables that provide insight into an organism's relationship to its environment.

Endophagy: The propensity of the female mosquito to take a blood meal inside a human dwelling.

Endophily: The propensity of the female mosquito to rest inside a human dwelling after taking a blood meal.

Exophagy: The propensity of the female mosquito to take a blood meal outdoors.

Exophily: The propensity of the female mosquito to rest outdoors after taking a blood meal.

Gametocytes: The final stage in the lifecycle of the malaria parasite. The female anopheline mosquito takes up these male and female forms of the parasite when she takes a blood meal from an infected host, and the gametocytes combine sexually in the mid-gut of the mosquito.

Holoendemicity: A state of year-round, heavy transmission of malaria. Malaria in holoendemic zones is stable, with rates of parasitemia continuously greater than 75 percent among children under 1 year of age and with spleen rates greater than 75 percent in the 2- to 9-year-old age cohort but low in adults. There is a considerable degree of effective immunity outside of the childhood years.

Hyperendemicity: A state of seasonal, intense transmission of malaria. Malaria in hyperendemic zones is often considered to be stable, characterized by rates of parasitemia continuously greater than 50 percent among children under 1 year of age and with spleen rates continuously greater than 50 percent in the 2- to 9-year-old age cohort and greater than 25 percent in adults. The degree of acquired immunity outside of the childhood years is lower than in holoendemic zones.

Hypoendemicity: A state of low transmission of malaria. Malaria in hypoendemic zones is characterized by rates of parasitemia of 10 percent or less among children aged 2–9 years and with spleen rates of 10 percent or less in the same cohort. The degree of acquired immunity is low.

Mesoendemicity: A state of seasonal, unstable transmission of malaria. Malaria in mesoendemic zones is characterized by rates of parasitemia of between 11 and 50 percent among children aged 2–9 years and with spleen rates of between 11 and 50 percent in the same cohort. The degree of acquired immunity outside of the childhood years is lower than in hyperendemic zones.

Parasitemia: The state of parasitization of the human bloodstream. Asymptomatic infections involve latent parasitemia.

Protozoa: A phylum or group of phyla that contain single-celled microscopic animals with a defined nucleus. The malaria parasites are protozoa (rather than bacteria or viruses).

Quinine: The first disease-specific drug in the western *materia medica*. It is an alkaloid that is isolated from the bark of the cinchona tree.

Sporozoite: The final form of the malaria parasite that develops within the female anopheline mosquito and is injected from the mosquito's salivary glands when she takes a blood meal.

Vector capacity: The ability of the infected female mosquito to transmit the parasite, which is determined by a number of variables, including zoophily. If a female anopheline mosquito infected with a human malaria parasite takes a blood meal from another animal, the sporozoites injected during the blood meal are unable to complete their lifecycle.

Vector competence: The ability of the female mosquito to host a parasite. The lifespans of some anopheline species are shortened after infection by the parasites. Some anopheline species have immune systems that are largely competent to prevent infection by the parasites. Other anopheline species have evolved to host the parasites without incurring major fitness costs.

Zoonoses: Diseases that have their origins in nonhuman animal species and that jump species barriers to infect human beings.

Zoophily: The propensity of the female of mosquito species to prefer a blood meal from an animal species other than *Homo sapiens sapiens* (human beings). These propensities vary among anopheline species and are an important determinant of vector capacity to transmit malaria.

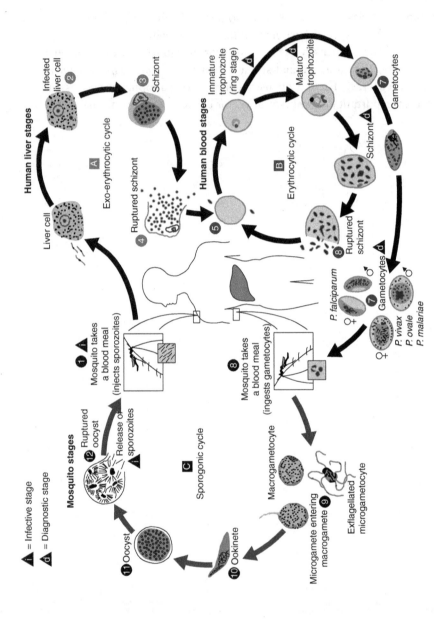

The Lifecycle of the Malaria Parasite
Adapted from the CDC website: http://www.cdc.gov/malaria/about/biology

An Introduction to African Malaria

Malaria is one of the most important infectious diseases in tropical Africa. It ignites 100–200 million bouts of illness annually, most mild and some severe. It kills by current estimates around 650,000 to 1.2 million Africans every year. Although there is no agreement on the best methodology for determining the number of malaria deaths – and thus the wide range of estimated mortality – specialists agree that the annual deaths are lower than those of just a few years ago.[1] A campaign to promote the use of bed nets, spray insecticides on the interior walls of dwellings, and provide antimalarial drugs is driving the numbers down.

Malaria has been an epidemiologically significant disease in tropical Africa for many millennia. Today, tropical Africa is the global epicenter of malarial infections. Malariologists estimate that approximately 90 percent of all malaria deaths occur in tropical Africa. The parasites that cause malaria and the mosquitoes that transmit the parasites are under assault, yet the infections are tenacious, and the dynamics of transmission are complex, volatile, and difficult to extinguish. Into the foreseeable future, malaria will remain a heavy disease burden under which Africans work and raise families.

---

[1] For the lower estimate, see World Health Organization, World Malaria Report 2011 (Geneva: World Health Organization, 2011). Available online: http://www.who.int/malaria/world_malaria_report_2011/en (accessed 15 May 2013). For the higher estimate, see Christopher J. L. Murray, Lisa C. Rosenfeld, Stephen S. Lim, Kathryn G. Andrews, Kyle J. Foreman, Diana Haring, Nancy Fullman, Mohsen Naghavi, Rafael Lozano, and Alan D. Lopez, "Global Malaria Mortality Between 1980 and 2010: A Systematic Analysis," *The Lancet*, vol. 379, no. 9814, 4 February 2012, 413–431.

THE EVOLUTION OF THE MALARIAL ENVIRONMENTS

On the basis of microbiological evidence and genetic studies, the broad picture of early human malarial infections is coming into focus.[2] Human beings have long been afflicted by several different species of one-celled parasites known as *plasmodia* that cause human malaria, and it is likely that four of the five species (*Plasmodium vivax, P. falciparum, P. malariae*, and *P. ovale*) originated in tropical Africa, the birthplace of ancient humankind.[3] This malaria burden was probably very light during the early epochs of gathering, fishing, and scavenging, when our ancestors traveled in small bands and had only infrequent contacts with others. The earliest infections were zoonotic: they were transferred by species of mosquitoes that belonged to the genus *Anopheles*, which took blood meals from great apes who were infected by simian malarias and which then bit humans. The frequent displacements of early human groups typically meant that they moved beyond the flight range of the anopheline mosquitoes and thus that ongoing transmission of the parasites was rare.

One hundred thousand years ago – and perhaps even earlier – our ancestors began to settle along the banks of tropical African waterways to fish and to socialize during a few months of the year. These early camps provided a new epidemiological setting that facilitated a seasonal pattern of transmission of the malaria parasites.

---

[2] For an exploration of this early history, see James L. A. Webb, Jr., *Humanity's Burden: A Global History of Malaria* (New York: Cambridge University Press, 2009), 18–41.

[3] On falciparum, see Weimin Liu, Yingling Li, Gerald H. Learn, Rebecca S. Rudicell, Joel D. Robertson, Brandon F. Keele, Jean-Bosco N. Ndjango, Crickette M. Sanz, David B. Morgan, Sabrina Locatelli, Mary K. Gonder, Philip J. Kranzusch, Peter D. Walsh, Eric Delaporte, Eitel Mpoudi-Ngole, Alexander V. Georgiev, Martin N. Muller, George M. Shaw, Martine Peeters, Paul M. Sharp, Julian C. Rayner, and Beatrice H. Hahn, "Origin of the Human Malaria Parasite *Plasmodium falciparum* in Gorillas," *Nature*, vol. 467, 23 September 2010, 420–425.

For divergent interpretations of the origins of vivax, see Richard Culleton and Richard Carter, "African *Plasmodium vivax*: Distribution and Origins," *International Journal for Parasitology*, vol. 42 (2012), 1091–1097; Jane M. Carlton, Ararup Das, and Ananias A. Escalante, "Genomics, Population Genetics and Evolutionary History of *Plasmodium vivax*," *Advances in Parasitology*, vol. 81 (2013), 203–222.

Recently, researchers have discovered that a fifth species, *P. knowlesi*, infects human beings. Its distribution is limited to Southeast Asia. See Janet Cox-Singh and Balbir Singh, "Knowlesi Malaria: Newly Emergent and of Public Health Importance?," *Trends in Parasitology*, vol. 24, no. 9 (2008), 406–410.

For a graphic representation of the lifecycle of the malaria parasite, see page xxii.

The parasites caused disease.[4] In the case of vivax, malariae, and the relatively rare ovale infections, the disease frequently took the form of high fevers interspersed with chills, accompanied by nausea and diarrhea. It frequently produced anemia and an accompanying debilitation. These afflictions made it difficult to participate in the activities essential to group survival. Vivax emerged as the most important early malarial burden because the parasite had evolved with a dormant phase that allowed it to re-emerge from the liver after months or even years, and thus new rounds of infection were not dependent on the misfortune of the occasional cross-species infection.[5] The burden of vivax over time was sufficiently heavy to select for a human genetic variation that mitigated the damage.

The critical genetic mutation took place in a surface antigen on the hemoglobin molecule. The mutation, known as Duffy Red Blood Cell antigen negativity – or Duffy negativity, was spectacularly successful. It prevented the parasite from infecting the red blood cell. The vivax parasite could not cause disease, and it could not reproduce. Duffy negativity was a definitive dead end for the vivax parasite.

Today, Duffy negativity is widely distributed in tropical Africa (see Map I.1). Its distribution probably reflects its early emergence tens of thousands of years ago and the competitive reproductive advantage of freedom from vivax infections and relapses enjoyed by those who carried the mutation. In a profound sense, the expanding expression of Duffy negativity was *the* determinative influence on the nature of African malaria. Vivax, the most common malaria parasite outside of tropical Africa, is rare in tropical Africa today.[6] Paradoxically, although Duffy negativity prevents vivax infections without health costs to the bearer, there have been enormous indirect costs borne by virtually everyone in tropical Africa.

---

[4] I use a shorthand when referring to an infection or disease caused by a malaria parasite: for example, a "falciparum infection" refers to an infection caused by *P. falciparum*.

[5] Ovale also developed a dormant liver phase. Relapsing ovale infections, in contrast to relapsing vivax infections, are often asymptomatic; the asexual parasite count rarely reaches high density; and the course of parasitemia is short compared to the other malaria parasite that cause sickness in humans. [William E. Collins and Geoffrey M. Jeffery, "*Plasmodium ovale*: Parasite and Disease," *Clinical Microbiology Reviews*, vol. 18, no. 3 (2005), 574, 578.]

[6] Vivax infections are transmitted among the small percentage of the population that is not protected by the Duffy mutation. See Franck Prugnolle, Virginie Rougeron, Pierre Becquart, Antoine Berry, Boris Makanga, Nil Rahola, Céline Arnathau, Barthélémy Ngoubangoye, Sandie Menard, Eric Willaume, Francisco J. Ayala, Didier Fontenille, Benjamin Ollomo, Patrick Durand, Christophe Paupy, and François Renaud, "Diversity, Host Switching and Evolution of *Plasmodium vivax* Infecting Great Apes," *Proceedings of the National Academy of Sciences*, vol. 110, no. 20 (2013), 8123–8128.

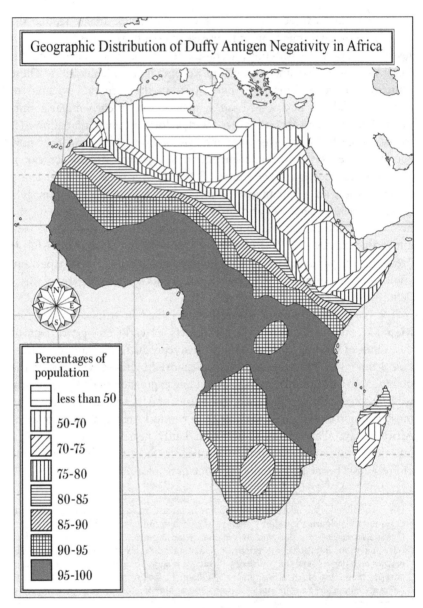

Geographic Distribution of Duffy Antigen Negativity in Africa

Percentages of population

- less than 50
- 50-70
- 70-75
- 75-80
- 80-85
- 85-90
- 90-95
- 95-100

MAP I.I. Geographic Distribution of Duffy Antigen Negativity in Africa
Adapted from L. Luca Cavalli-Sforza, Paolo Menozzi, and Alberto Piazza. *The History and Geography of Human Genes* (Princeton, NJ: Princeton University Press, 1994), genetic maps, 160. The data codings for Madagascar are derived from a map entitled "The Spatial Distribution of the Duffy Negative Phenotype Map in 2010 in Madagascar" made by the Malaria Atlas Project. Available online: http://www.map.ox.ac.uk/browse-resources/duffy-negativity/duffy-negativity/MDG/

Elsewhere in the global tropics, falciparum and vivax infections exist in a very rough equilibrium, jostling with one another as the locally or regionally dominant cause of malarial infection. (*P. malariae* generally plays a minor role; *P. ovale*, restricted to West Africa and the Pacific, is an infection of even lesser significance; and *P. knowlesi* is rare and restricted to Southeast Asia.) Tropical Africa is the grand exception. The near exclusion of vivax malaria from tropical Africa via the spread of Duffy negativity allowed for the broad dominance of falciparum malaria.[7] This constituted an epidemiological disaster. The African mosaics of malaria parasites came to be dominated by falciparum, the most dangerous parasite.

Falciparum infections, like those caused by the vivax, malariae, and ovale parasites, ignite a characteristic pattern of fever and chills with nausea and diarrhea and produce anemia. Falciparum infections, however, frequently cause more dire complications. Falciparum malaria can involve temporary or permanent coma, mental retardation, organ failure, and death. Falciparum, in the absence of medical intervention, may kill up to 20 percent of nonimmune individuals who are infected in the course of an epidemic.[8] By comparison, the death toll of vivax malaria is dramatically lower. Vivax, in the absence of medical intervention, may kill 1 or 2 percent of nonimmune individuals who are newly infected, and up to 5 percent in the case of individuals with a compromised nutritional or immunological status. No mortality estimates have been developed for malariae or ovale in tropical Africa, in part because these infections often occur in combination with falciparum.

Falciparum parasites thus posed a greater threat to tropical Africans than did vivax, malariae, or ovale parasites. The early history of falciparum infections is currently under laboratory investigation. Recent research suggests that a significant increase in falciparum infections may have occurred about 40,000–20,000 years ago.[9] The microbiological responses

[7] The dynamics of mixed infections are complex and only partly modeled. Longitudinal studies of mixed infections are rare. Mixed vivax and falciparum infections, however, are estimated to result in a far lower rate of severe clinical malaria. See Daniel P. Mason and F. Ellis McKenzie, "Blood Stage Dynamics and Clinical Implications of Mixed Plasmodium Vivax-Plasmodium Falciparum Infections," *American Journal of Tropical Medicine and Hygiene*, vol. 61, no. 3 (1999), 367–374.

[8] J. -F. Trape and C. Rogier, "Combating Malaria Morbidity and Mortality by Reducing Transmission," *Parasitology Today*, vol. 12, no. 6 (1996), 239.

[9] Hsiao-Han Chang, Daniel J. Park, Kevin J. Galinsky, Stephen F. Schaffner, Douda Ndiaye, Omar Ndir, Souleymane Mboup, Roger C. Wiegand, Sarah K. Volkman, Pardis C. Sabeti, Dyann F. Wirth, Daniel E. Neafsey, and Daniel L. Hartl, "Genomic Sequencing of

6   The Long Struggle Against Malaria in Tropical Africa

to heavy falciparum pressure, however, appear to have occurred in a more recent historical era. Falciparum may have begun to exert heavy selection pressure with the development of paracultivation of yams in the woodlands and forest-edge ecologies within the last 10,000–15,000 years. This falciparum pressure selected for genetic mutations that would convey a survival advantage, as vivax pressure had done in an earlier epoch.

Unlike Duffy negativity, however, the genetic hemoglobin mutations to falciparum pressure, known as *thalassemias*, conveyed significant costs as well as benefits. The bearers of these thalassemias can suffer severe anemia, growth failure, jaundice, and other complications. In tropical Africa, the mutation known as alpha-thalassemia is widespread. One of its most common variants is known as the sickle-cell trait, because it produces a sickle-shaped deformation of the red blood cell. These mutations are inherited, and when both parents biologically pass on the mutated gene, and thus the child is homozygous for the mutation, the health burden is great. Most children in tropical Africa who are homozygous for the sickle-cell trait do not live to the age of sexual maturity. Children who are heterozygous (with one mutated gene and one normal gene) inherit some protection from severe malaria.[10]

Plasmodium falciparum Malaria Parasites from Senegal Reveals the Demographic History of the Population," *Molecular Biology Evolution*, vol. 29, no. 11 (2012), 4327–4339.

[10] The normal hemoglobin molecule is made up of four chains of proteins, two alpha-globin and two beta-globin. The genetic mutations to malaria pressure involve changes in one or more of the genes that govern the production of these proteins. Hemoglobin S is a mutation caused by a particular amino acid substitution in the beta chain (valine for glutamic acid at position 6). For a brief overview of red cell polymorphisms and malaria, see Kevin Marsh, "Immunology of Malaria," in David A. Warrell and Herbert M. Gilles (eds.), *Essential Malariology* (London: Arnold Publishers, 2002), 253–256.

The thalassemias are a heterogenous group of conditions characterized by a reduced rate of production of one or more of the globin chains. In tropical Africa, the principal mutations are in the alpha-globin protein. For evidence of the protective value of alpha thalassemia, see Frank P. Mockenhaupt, Stephan Ehrhardt, Sabine Gellert, Rowland N. Otchwemah, Ekkehart Dietz, Sylvester D. Anemana, and Ulrich Bienzle, "Alpha +–thalassemia Protects African Children from Severe Malaria," *Blood*, vol. 104, no. 7 (2004), 2003–2006.

For the distribution and gene frequency of the alpha-globin mutations, see L. Luca Cavalli-Sforza, Paolo Menozzi, and Alberto Piazza, *The History and Geography of Human Genes* (Princeton, NJ: Princeton University Press, 1994), figures 2.14.5.A [world distribution] and 2.14.5.B [African distribution], 150; for world distribution of the beta-globin mutation, figure 2.14.6.B, 151.

It is possible that the hemoglobin mutation known as Hemoglobin C affords protection against malaria, although expert opinions differ. For the distribution and gene frequency of Hemoglobin C in Africa, see Cavalli-Sforza, et al., *History and Geography of the Human Genes*, figure 2.14.2, 148.

Over thousands of years, apparently well after the emergence and spread of Duffy negativity, as Africans extended their settlements throughout the continent, they carried malaria parasites with them in their blood (Map I.2). These were long-unfolding processes launched from West and Northeast Africa. The population movements from West Africa are known as the *Bantu migrations*; Christopher Ehret has analyzed the close connections between the languages spoken by the modern descendants of the original agricultural migrants and has argued for the relatively recent nature of the two-phase expansion, dated to 5500–4500 BCE and 1500 BCE–500 CE. From northeast Africa, the southward and westward movements of pastoralists and farmers known as the *Cushitic migrations* are dated to 4000–3000 BCE. Some of these pioneers reached southern Africa only in the early centuries of the second millennium CE.[11] There, agriculturalists and "mixed farmers," who practiced both agriculture and livestock herding, displaced hunting and gathering peoples and established new malarial environments. Even within long-settled zones, as African communities slowly built their numbers, they transformed their environments. In a broad sense, human communities inaugurated and/or intensified the malarial environments. In the forested zones, they cut holes in the forest canopy in order to grow food and inadvertently created new mosquito habitat. In the practices of vegeculture and seed-based agriculture, they created new contours to capture rainwater and created mosquito-breeding habitats. In building huts and compounds, they used local soils dug from "borrow-pits" that then filled with rainwater and in which mosquitoes bred. By settling, they improved the prospects for mosquitoes searching for blood meals in order to reproduce, and over time, the human settlements facilitated the evolution of anopheline species that had a strong preference for taking blood meals from humans rather than other animals. In these respects, the malarial environments of tropical Africa are relatively recent artifacts of human settlement.

As populations grew, societies became more complex. The tropical malarial environments, once highly localized, became increasingly integrated, with regional variations. This was true in all of the ecological zones – the sahel, savanna, woodland, lake coast, seacoast, and forest. In all zones, the parasite mosaics were dominated by falciparum. The environments differed in the intensity of transmission by virtue of the ecological behaviors of the different anopheline species that had adapted to the

---

[11] Christopher Ehret, *The Civilizations of Africa: A History to 1800* (Charlottesville: University of Virginia Press, 2002).

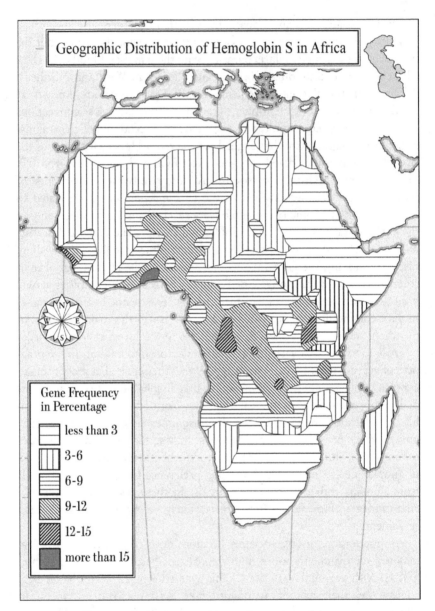

MAP 1.2. Geographic Distribution of Hemoglobin S in Africa
Adapted from L. Luca Cavalli-Sforza, Paolo Menozzi, and Alberto Piazza. *The History and Geography of Human Genes* (Princeton, NJ: Princeton University Press, 1994), figure 2.14.1.D, 147.

vegetation covers, patterns of rainfall, and the available blood meals in the regional habitats.

There were also important variations by altitude. Temperature was a principal limiting factor for both mosquitoes and human beings. In most highland regions above 6,500 feet, anopheline mosquitoes were rare, and the temperatures were typically too low to allow the parasites to reproduce. Settled human communities at these altitudes were sparse too, because cooler temperatures reduced the productivity of agriculture. Below 6,500 feet, the highland regions varied considerably, according to differences in physical relief, vegetation, and agricultural practices, but communities located between 3,500 and 6,500 feet altitude could be subject to occasional epidemics.[12] Humidity was also a limiting factor: to the north of the sahel, the environment was too dry to permit agriculture, and in the full desert, the transmission of malaria was limited to oasis settlements. There, the arrival of long-distance traders who had picked up infections elsewhere could set off an outbreak among oasis dwellers.

Parasite Mosaics

As falciparum became the dominant parasite in the regional configurations or *mosaics*, the *P. falciparum* parasite mutated into an array of different genotypes. The genotypes within a given mosaic played a central role in infections. During early encounters, African children acquired specific immunities through exposure to one or more of the genotypes. Cross-immunity between genotypes, however, was imperfect, and when a child or adult struggled with a new genotype for the first time, a severe bout of disease typically ensued.

The parasite mosaics in tropical Africa were unstable. Over millennia, African pioneers expanded into all of the ecological zones of the subcontinent and founded new communities. African merchants in trade diasporas carried goods across long distances, linking communities in different ecological zones. During the precolonial centuries before European military conquest of tropical Africa (1879–1914), predatory raiding and warfare between African states engulfed many African communities. Large numbers of people were forced to migrate within tropical Africa, and many were captured and sold as slaves. These internal slave trades, in

---

[12] Jean Mouchet, Pierre Carnevale, Marc Coosemans, Jean Julvez, Sylvie Manguin, Dominique Richard-Lenoble, and Jacques Sircoulon, *Biodiversité du paludisme dans le monde* (Montrouge: Éditions John Libbey Eurotext, 2004), 81–82.

conjunction with the chaotic displacement of populations during times of political and economic upheaval, brought about an unprecedented, rapid mixing of the parasite genotypes.

This was true as well of the external slave trades that brought captives into unfamiliar disease environments and thereby extended and reconfigured the parasite mosaics. This was the case, for example, during the long centuries of the external slave trades when many millions left tropical Africa in chains, sold into forced labor in North Africa, the Indian Ocean world, and the Americas. The Atlantic slave trade was the last of the three great outflows of African captives, and it is the best documented: during the seventeenth, eighteenth, and nineteenth centuries, the volume of slave exports into the Americas far outstripped those to other external markets. In the New World, the forcible transfer of some 12 million Africans transformed disease environments, creating lethal falciparum-rich malarial stews in the Caribbean and in regions of the South Atlantic fringe where African populations were in the majority.[13]

The parasitological details of these historical processes are not recoverable using current techniques. The broad picture within tropical Africa, however, is reasonably clear, with two salient features. First, in areas in which Duffy negativity was widely expressed – in all of tropical Africa – *P. falciparum* dominated the subcontinental mosaic and, by the early twentieth century, was involved in more than 90 percent of all malarial infections.[14] Second, many malarial infections involved more than one species of parasite, and most mixed infections involved *P. malariae*.[15] The usual peak prevalence of *P. malariae* in the parasite mosaics studied

---

[13] Webb, *Humanity's Burden*, 66–91; John R. McNeill, *Mosquito Empires: Ecology and War in the Greater Caribbean, 1620–1914* (New York: Cambridge University Press, 2010).

[14] The first studies of African parasites held that falciparum infections were the only kind to be found among the African communities of the west coast of the continent. Stephens and Christophers, on the basis of an analysis of 639 cases, found not a single vivax or malariae parasite and judged that they were nonexistent. [J. W. W. Stephens and S. R. Christophers, "The Malarial Infection of Native Children," in *Reports to the Malaria Committee of the Royal Society*, third series (London, 1900), 4–5.]

[15] In the wider world, malariae was far less common an infection than vivax, and among malariologists working outside of tropical Africa, it received little research attention. [Émile Marchoux, "La fièvre quarte et son mystère," *Revue coloniale de médecine et chirurgie*, 15 October 1930, 213–220.]

From the earliest investigations of parasite prevalence in clinical malaria, most findings agreed on the predominance of falciparum parasites and that *P. malariae*, which caused the distinctive seventy-two-hour fever known as *quartan malaria*, was the second most prevalent malaria parasite. Because malariae was far less lethal than falciparum, it attracted far less attention.

in the early twentieth century was on the order of 15–30 percent, although it could occasionally exceed this range. Malariae infections seem to have increased during the dry seasons and have been suppressed by more frequent falciparum infections during the wet seasons. Malariae was far milder than falciparum, and it is estimated to have produced relatively little severe illness, perhaps only 1–2 percent of clinical fever episodes.[16]

During the era of European colonialism, the introduction of infected military troops from outside of tropical Africa transformed some of the local parasite mosaics. In Freetown, for example, malariologists discovered an epidemic of malariae infections that began in the late 1920s. It was likely the result of a new malariae strain introduced via troop transports during the First World War. According to their studies, malariae infections increased at the expense of falciparum infections, and they occurred in greater frequency in children over the age of 3 and with the highest prevalence between the ages of 5 and 9.[17] In 1935, the largest percentage of childhood infections – some 60 percent – was still malariae.[18] This may have been near its peak. By 1940, the malariae rate had dropped to 11.4 percent and by 1942 to 0.4 percent.[19]

Vectors and the Transmission of Malaria

The parasite mosaics constitute an important dimension of the changing malarial environments of tropical Africa. Even more significant from an epidemiological point of view are the dynamic changes in the distribution and density of the species of *Anopheles* mosquitoes that hosted and transmitted the malaria parasites.[20] There are three major species of

[16] Ivo Mueller, Peter A. Zimmerman, and John C. Reeder, "*Plasmodium malariae* and *Plasmodium ovale* – the 'Bashful' Malaria Parasites," *Trends in Parasitology*, vol. 23, no. 6 (2007), 278–283.

[17] R. M. Gordon and T. H. Davey, "*P. malariae* in Freetown, Sierra Leone," *Annals of Tropical Medicine and Parasitology*, vol. 26 (1932), 65–84; R. M. Gordon and T. H. Davey, "A Further Note on the Increase of *P. malariae* in Freetown, Sierra Leone," *Annals of Tropical Medicine and Parasitology*, vol. 27 (1933), 53–55.

[18] H. Peaston and E. A. Renner, "Report on an Examination of the Spleen- and Parasite-Rates in School Children in Freetown, Sierra, Leone," *Annals of Tropical Medicine and Parasitology*, vol. 33 (1939), 49–59.

[19] John Storey, "A Review of Malaria Work in Sierra Leone, 1900–1964," *West African Medical Journal*, vol. 21, no. 3 (1972), 58–59, 62. The malarial exchanges were not unidirectional. During the First World War, South Africans and New Zealanders came down with falciparum during their stopovers in Freetown.

[20] The outstanding encyclopedic work on the global biodiversity of malaria is Jean Mouchet et al., *Biodiversité du paludisme dans le monde*.

"super-transmitters": *An. gambiae sensu stricto*, *An. arabiensis*, and *An. funestus*.[21] They flitted throughout the continent, and one or more were present across all ecological zones from desert-edge to dense rainforest, from the lowlands to the moderate highlands, and in virtually all ecological niches. They were not alone. Other anopheline mosquitoes, such as *An. nili*, *An. moucheti*, *An. melas*, *An. mascariensis*, and *An. paludi* were highly significant regional vectors with narrower ranges. Many other anopheline species with lesser competencies to host the parasite and lesser capacities to transmit malaria were regional or local vectors of consequence, if only in secondary or tertiary roles.[22]

The females of these anopheline species took blood meals from humans and other animals in order to have nutrients for their eggs to develop, and in the act of drawing blood, the infected female mosquitoes injected malaria parasites. There were, however, significant differences in the capacities of the vectors to transmit malaria that reflected a broad range of variables, including distinct biological endowments and behaviors in different ecological zones. Some vector species are remarkably adaptable and can thrive in a variety of zones. Others cannot. The mosquitoes of some vector species have guts in which the parasites have difficulty reproducing, and the mosquitoes of other species may get sick while hosting the parasites.[23] Some species have longer lifespans in cooler weather, and in cooler weather the metabolism of the parasites slows down and the incubation period in the mosquito is extended. Some vectors have a strong biting preference for humans. Others do not have a preference for one type

---

[21] In the first chapters of this book that deal with the first half of the twentieth century, I use the term *Anopheles gambiae* to refer to the species complex; the malariological reports of the era do not allow for greater precision. In the chapters that deal with the second half of the twentieth century, I will refer to the individual anopheline species (e.g., *Anopheles gambiae sensu stricto [s.s.]* and *Anopheles arabiensis*) and to the species complex as *Anopheles gambiae sensu lato [s.l.]*.

   An. funestus sensu stricto will be referred to in this book simply as *An. funestus*. It, too, was part of a broader grouping. The other sibling species of the funestus species complex, however, feed exclusively on animals other than human beings and thus have no role in human malaria transmission.

[22] Some of the species are identical in appearance and, until the development of advanced biological technologies, were held to be a single species. For a list of significant vectors in tropical Africa, see Mouchet et al., *Biodiversité du paludisme*, 67.

[23] Mosquitoes that do get sick live shorter lives and thus are less efficient at transmitting malaria, although this is difficult to document. Mosquito sickness has been documented in laboratory conditions in which the parasite load is very high; most mosquitoes that transmit malaria have far lighter parasite loads. Personal communication from Richard Pollack, May 2013.

of blood source over another. Because the parasites that cause human malaria can only complete their lifecycle within the human organism, whenever mosquitoes inject the malaria parasites into nonhuman animals, the parasites encounter a dead end.[24]

Biologists generally represent these interacting ecological variables as part of a natural system of dynamics known as *bionomics*. This is a highly useful approach in that it allows for the measurement and study of the interaction of a discrete set of variables. But from an epidemiological point of view, bionomics is of more limited utility because it does not take into account the influence of human cultural practices on malaria transmission. To cite two simple examples: if people sit around smoky fires in the evening, they receive fewer mosquito bites; if people sleep outdoors rather than indoors, they will receive more mosquito bites. In order to get a fuller idea of the epidemiological realities, it is necessary to span the chasm between the natural sciences and the social sciences.

Acquired Immunity

Tropical Africa remains the most challenging disease environment in the world, owing to the burden of vector-borne and water-borne diseases. Malaria, in league with a spate of bacterial and viral infections, has threatened the ability of African communities to increase their numbers. Malaria steals away infants, toddlers, and children who are just reaching the age of useful labor. The malaria toll continues to be paid in some communities even by their adolescents. For many African communities, the death rates among the very young are still extremely high in the early twenty-first century.[25]

The consequences of childhood falciparum malaria infections range widely. Many infants are partially protected for several months by the

[24] The principal exception to this generalization is that of *P. knowlesi*, which can reproduce in both long-tailed macaques and human beings. This parasite, as noted earlier, is not transmitted in tropical Africa.

[25] These high death rates may have played a role in the evolution of some African communities' conceptions of childhood and childhood agency. In the West African communities studied by the anthropologist Alma Gottlieb, for example, infants were held to be ancestors from the afterlife. The role of the "parents" was to determine the wishes of the ancestors/infants, and an early departure back into the afterlife – that is, the death of the infant – was understood to be an expression of free will on the part of the infant that was not to be struggled against. Alma Gottlieb, *The Afterlife Is Where We Come From: The Culture of Infancy in West Africa* (Chicago: University of Chicago Press, 2004).

transfer in utero of protective substances from the mother and/or by breastfeeding. Many endure bouts of malaria and thrive. Some die within days or suffer life-long disabilities as a result of cerebral malaria that impairs mental abilities. Some suffer the decreased functioning of internal organs. Some experience a general deterioration of health. These costs are in addition to health complications that accrue to some bearers of the hemoglobin mutations that help to protect against the worst ravages of falciparum malaria.

All who survive, including those who suffer impairments of one type or another, receive some level of protection from the dire consequences of future bouts of malaria. Researchers distinguish between three types of this acquired or adaptive immunity: (1) antidisease immunity, which confers protection against clinical disease associated with a given parasite density; (2) antiparasite immunity, which protects against parasitemia by affecting the density of parasites in the blood; and (3) premunition, which maintains a low-grade and generally asymptomatic parasitemia and thereby protects against the clinical manifestations of new infections. This complexity is generally referred to collectively as *acquired immunity*. It is very hard won, and it is a precious asset in an environment in which an individual may receive a large number of bites from parasitized mosquitoes – in some areas up to several hundred or more infective bites per year.[26]

The degree of immunity from malarial disease varies greatly. This is in part a function of the intensity of transmission. In areas where the levels of parasite transmission are very high – on the order of several hundred infective bites or more per year – the level of protective immunity is correspondingly high. In these areas, some individuals who are infected repeatedly can be utterly asymptomatic. Heavy parasite infections can co-exist with general good health. It is thus easily understandable that among these communities there are many who think malaria is not a serious problem. The members of communities in which the level of transmission intensity is lower tend to have less robust levels of protective immunity. Partial immunity, nonetheless, is still a profound boon. Partial immunity protects from the worst ravages of the infections, and most individuals with partial immunity, when infected, suffer relatively mild flu-like symptoms.

---

[26] For a detailed introduction to acquired immunity, see Denise L. Doolan, Carlato Dobaño, and J. Kevin Baird, "Acquired Immunity to Malaria," *Clinical Microbiology Reviews*, vol. 22, no. 1 (2009), 13–36.

In global terms, the acquisition at a population level of immunity to falciparum infection is distinctively African. There are other peoples – in coastal New Guinea, for example – who have similar immunities, but nowhere outside of tropical Africa is there a large landmass in which the acquisition of immunity to malaria is a defining feature of population health.

European Vulnerability

The intense transmission of falciparum malaria in tropical Africa had long helped structure its trade relations and cultural exchanges with the wider world. When caravan traders from North Africa crossed the Sahara and entered the savannas, or when maritime traders from the Arabian Peninsula, Persian Gulf, the Mediterranean, or North Atlantic landed on the seacoasts of tropical Africa, they encountered a new and hostile epidemiological environment. Falciparum malaria killed many of the non-immune foreigners who dared to engage in African commerce.

These mortality costs were so high that historians credit the disease environment of tropical Africa with "protecting" the subcontinent from direct colonization during the era of the slave trades. Along the oceanic and desert frontiers of tropical Africa, the long-term pattern was for male merchants who survived the disease challenges to establish liaisons with indigenous women and to contribute to mixed cultural communities. Swahili communities, with their distinctive mixture of Arab and Black African ("Bantu") culture, and Luso-African communities formed on the eastern coast. Luso-African, Franco-African, Anglo-African, and other blends of European and Black African culture took shape along the western coast.[1]

During the centuries of the Atlantic slave trade, death rates among European traders and sailors who dropped anchor off the western African coasts seeking slaves, gold, or tropical agricultural products were exceedingly high, particularly for those who jumped ship to seek their fortunes in coastal trading communities or for those soldiers whose

---

[1] James L. A. Webb, Jr., "Malaria in Africa," *History Compass*, vol. 9, no. 3 (2011), 162–170.

misfortune it was to be stationed in a coastal European fort. Malaria, along with yellow fever, exacted an appalling price from the floating and resident European communities and earned for tropical Africa its designation as "the white man's grave."[2]

The malarial risks to Europeans along the West African coast remained extremely dire until the adoption of an antimalarial prophylaxis in the mid-nineteenth century. The sailors and traders who downed a daily ration of bitter wine infused with the medically active alkaloids of cinchona bark – the first disease-specific medication in the Western *materia medica* – reduced their vulnerability to this deadly fever. In the event of a serious attack, additional treatments with quinine, or with other alkaloids in powdered cinchona bark, if administered in time, stood a good chance of fending off the worst. Yet the magic of the bark, owing to adulteration or under-dosage, could be as ephemeral as stardust. Europeans suffered an ongoing toll of malarial fevers and deaths.

EPIDEMIOLOGICAL INTEGRATION

Africans also suffered from a historic collision with exotic pathogens. During the centuries of the export slave trades, tropical Africans had borne a share of the brunt of the epidemiological integration with other world regions.[3] Traders from Europe, North Africa, and South Asia inadvertently brought with them an array of pathogens, and some of these new diseases must have had the potential to spread beyond the coastal communities into the interior of the continent. During the second half of the nineteenth century, as the eastern coastal regions of the continent were drawn increasingly into international commerce, and as the slave trades then reached into Central Africa from both the eastern and western coasts, this integration accelerated. Cholera epidemics, ignited by the introduction of a lethal bacillus from South Asia, struck.[4] From South

---

[2] Philip D. Curtin, "Epidemiology and the Slave Trade," *Political Science Quarterly*, vol. 83, no. (1968), 190–216; K. G. Davies, "The Living and the Dead: White Mortality in West Africa, 1684–1732," in Stanley L. Engerman and Eugene D. Genovese (eds.), *Race and Slavery in the Western Hemisphere: Quantitative Studies* (Princeton: Princeton University Press, 1975), 83–98; Philip D. Curtin, *Death by Migration: Europe's Encounter with the Tropical World in the Nineteenth Century* (New York: Cambridge University Press, 1989).

[3] On the transfer of malaria from tropical Africa to the Americas, see Webb, *Humanity's Burden*, 66–91. On yellow fever, McNeill, *Mosquito Empires*.

[4] Myron Echenberg, *Africa in the Time of Cholera: A History of Pandemics from 1817 to the Present* (New York: Cambridge University Press, 2011).

America, the sand flea (*Tunga penetrans*) arrived via sailing ships and set off an epidemic of tungiasis, or foot and leg rot, which progressed from West Central Africa laterally across the continent.[5]

The most devastating event in this epochal process of epidemiological integration was the introduction in 1881 by the Italians into the Horn of Africa of the cattle epizootic known as *rinderpest*. The disease ripped through the bovine populations in Eritrea and Ethiopia and, over time, spread thousands of miles south, destroying approximately 90 percent of the livestock of pastoralists and mixed farming communities, causing the collapse of pastoral economies and widespread human starvation.[6]

In the context of this late-nineteenth-century epidemiological crisis, the malarial infections of adult Africans with some degree of acquired immunity receded to the status of a minor burden. Novel and frightening afflictions eclipsed the familiar toll of childhood malarial deaths and adult illnesses. The unfolding epidemiological crisis ran parallel with a profound realignment in the political economy of Atlantic trade that was to transform Africa's relationship with Europe.

THE TRAUMA OF CONQUEST

By the 1860s, the coastal markets of tropical Africa were in full transition from the trade in human captives to trade in "legitimate" goods.[7] The long abolitionist struggle to end the Atlantic slave trade and abolish the institution of slavery in the Americas had achieved notable successes, and European traders began to concentrate their efforts on the purchase of goods such as palm oil and palm kernel oil in western Africa and cloves and

---

[5] Helge Kjekshus, *Ecology Control and Economic Development in East African History* (Athens: Ohio University Press, 1996), 126–160.

[6] On rinderpest broadly, see C. A. Spinage, *Cattle Disease: A History* (New York: Springer Publishing, 2003). On southern Africa, Pule Phoofolo, "Epidemics and Revolutions: The Rinderpest Epidemic in Late Nineteenth Century Southern Africa," *Past and Present*, vol. 138, no. 1 (1993), 112–143.

[7] On the export of captives, see Philip D. Curtin, *The Atlantic Slave Trade: A Census* (Madison: University of Wisconsin Press, 1969).

    The decline in the export slave trade, however, did not signal the end of large-scale political violence within tropical Africa. Large conflicts convulsed African societies during the final decades of the century, including the Islamic jihads in western Africa and the expansion of warfare known as the *dificane* in eastern Africa. See Philip D. Curtin, Steven Feierman, Leonard Thompson, and Jan Vansina, *African History: From Earliest Times to Independence* (New York: Longman, 1995).

ivory in eastern Africa. Local African political authorities, merchants, and other owners of slaves responded by boosting production. The era of "legitimate trade" also inaugurated the establishment of new European commercial enterprises in many of the port towns of tropical Africa.

Beginning in 1879, European political authorities, whose national economies were locked in savage industrial competition with one another and suffering from a regional economic depression, launched campaigns in tropical Africa to stake out national territorial claims. They made alliances with some African states, brutally defeated the armies of other African states, and co-opted yet others. The "Scramble for Africa" called forth a new map of tropical Africa, with the boundaries of Portuguese, Spanish, German, Italian, Belgian, French, and British colonies inscribed on it. All but a handful of coastal polities with Euro-African communities already within the cultural and political orbit of European empires – and the colony of Liberia founded by African Americans from the United States – were swept up in the dramatic realignments.[8]

European officers directed the military campaigns, but African troops in European employ did most of the fighting in the Scramble for Africa. The health costs of keeping European troops in tropical Africa, even with the mid-century public health breakthroughs in water filtration and the sanitary disposal of human waste to reduce fecal-oral disease, remained high. Europeans were at high risk from vector-borne disease. Medical officers prescribed quinine, a cinchona alkaloid that was isolated chemically and marketed by pharmaceutical companies, for malaria prophylaxis. This reduced the European death toll, but malaria remained a major killer of European troops.

Dramatic political change across tropical Africa marked the last two decades of the nineteenth century. Across the western sahel, an Islamic jihadist movement reworked the political landscape. Large-scale political violence convulsed central Africa as Swahili Arab warlords clashed with regional African polities. In coastal West Africa, African intellectuals made the case for African rights and participation in civil governance and founded newspapers that gave them voice. Much political change, however, was initiated from abroad, as European industrial and commercial nations, seeking the possibility of economic advantage and fearing the prospects of disadvantage vis-à-vis their competitors, swept into tropical

---

[8] Thomas Pakenham, *The Scramble for Africa: White Man's Conquest of the Dark Continent from 1876–1912* (New York: Random House, 1991).

Africa and claimed its interior. Another regionally focused invasion proceeded from the interior of what is today the Republic of South Africa, near the southern frontier of tropical Africa, where miners discovered massive diamond fields in 1867 and massive gold deposits in 1886. These discoveries propelled European colonists north to search for additional sources of mineral wealth in the southern reaches of the tropical African malaria zone.[9] (See Map 1.1.)

As armies of conquest gave way to fledgling civil administrations, European missionaries, merchants, military men, government officials, prospecting miners, and land-seeking farmers filtered into the newly acquired colonial territories. The African environments were notoriously dangerous for whites, and the new arrivals sought recommendations about protection from malaria and other tropical diseases from "old Africa hands" with long experience and from books of medical advice.[10]

The Europeans had little interest in African antimalarial medicines for their own use.[11] In part, this was a function of the cultural disdain with which Europeans learned to judge Africans. Late-nineteenth-century European "science" taught that Africans were a less evolved race of humanity, and thus, by definition, most things African were deemed to be less advanced than were most things European. For many European administrators, traders, farmers, and missionaries in Africa, this was reason enough – along with the genuine difficulties of communication across the barriers of language and culture – for a general dismissal of the notion that African medical knowledge might have useful applications for themselves. Europeans, moreover, were blinded by what they could not see. Intensely aware of their own vulnerability to African fevers, they initially

---

[9] For an overview of nineteenth-century Africa, see Curtin et al., *African History*.

[10] See, for example, David Kerr Cross, *Health in Africa: A Medical Handbook for European Travellers and Residents, Embracing a Study of Malarial Fever as It Is Found in British Central Africa* (London: James Nisbet & Co., Ltd, 1897); and William Henry Crosse, *Hints, Suggestions and Medical Notes for Those Traveling in West Africa* (London: F. R. B. Parmeter, 1903).

[11] James L. A. Webb, Jr., "On Biomedicine, Transfers of Knowledge, and Malaria Treatments in Eastern North America and Tropical Africa," in David M. Gordon and Shepard Krech III (eds.), *Indigenous Knowledge and the Environment in Africa and North America* (Athens: Ohio University Press, 2012), 53–68.

The French botanist Auguste Chevalier (1873–1956) was an avid collector of African plants, and his research interests extended to African plant-based medicines. No African plant-based medicines, however, appear to have entered into the therapeutic antimalarial practices of Europeans. I am indebted to Tamara Giles-Vernick for bringing the little-studied research of Auguste Chevalier to my attention.

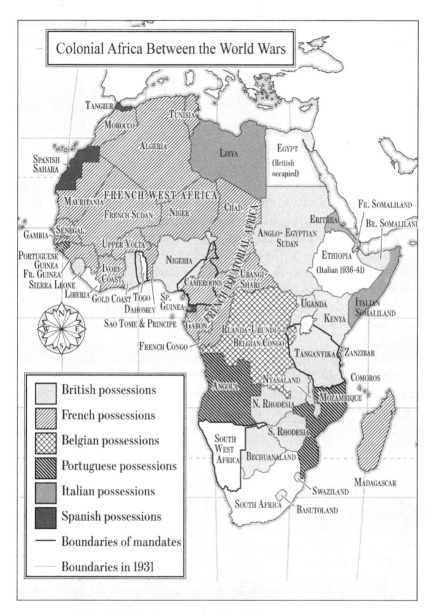

Colonial Africa Between the World Wars

British possessions

French possessions

Belgian possessions

Portuguese possessions

Italian possessions

Spanish possessions

— Boundaries of mandates

Boundaries in 1931

MAP 1.1. Colonial Africa Between the World Wars
Redrawn from Roland Oliver, *The African Experience* (New York: HarperCollins, 1991), 214.

judged that Africans were not. Europeans believed that they got malarial infections from other Europeans, and that there was a need to isolate Europeans with malarial fevers. The late-nineteenth-century European view was that, in tropical Africa, malaria was a problem of whites.[12]

THE EUROPEAN BARRIER DEFENSE: MOSQUITO NETTING

Early in the twentieth century, some Europeans in tropical Africa used mosquito netting to prevent buzzing mosquitoes and other insects from disturbing their sleep and as a barrier defense against malaria.[13] In principle, when hung from windows and across thresholds, mosquito netting blocked mosquitoes from entering the house. When hung over a bed, the mosquito netting worked by preventing mosquitoes from taking blood meals from people sleeping under it. The netting, however, impeded the flow of air and could be stiflingly hot to sleep under – particularly if the netting were made of muslin – and it was easily torn. Moreover, some of the mosquito netting available was too coarse to screen out the smaller anophelines, particularly *Anopheles funestus*, and in this case, even diligent usage would afford slight protection.[14]

Early in the twentieth century, investigative teams sent from the Liverpool School of Tropical Medicine to West Africa reported that Europeans frequently deployed their mosquito netting incompetently. As the team sent to Nigeria put it:

The mosquito curtain is astonishingly misused by Europeans on the West Coast of Africa. We very rarely met with one who used the curtains in a careful and proper manner. Almost all are so placed as to hang outside the bedposts and reach on to the ground, being either free or weighted. This is an improper way of hanging the curtains, which thus act as a trap for those mosquitoes which have taken shelter during the day-time under the bed – as very commonly happens. The majority of the nets were sometimes so torn as to be of no protective use whatever, others had a few holes. All these were practically useless – the persistent *Anopheles* will discover the smallest hole capable of affording its body admission in the search for blood. It

---

[12] For British perspectives on the differential vulnerability of whites to malaria, see Philip D. Curtin, *The Image of Africa: British Ideas and Action, 1780–1850* (Madison: University of Wisconsin Press, 1964); and Dennis G. Carlson, *African Fever: A Study of British Science, Technology, and Politics in West Africa, 1787–1864* (Canton, MA: Science History Publications, 1984).

[13] The buzzing mosquitoes of the genus *Culex* were far more abundant than the silent anophelines.

[14] C. W. Daniels, "Prophylaxis," in *Reports to the Malaria Committee of the Royal Society*, third series (London, 1900), 40.

was common to hear considerable surprise expressed at the presence of gorged mosquitoes inside these nets regularly every morning.[15]

THE EUROPEAN CHEMICAL DEFENSE: QUININE

Europeans also made use of quinine, an effective cure for malaria that had proved its worth for decades.[16] It was broadly considered to be a good defense against malarial infections and the best means of cure. Moreover, by the late nineteenth century, the price of quinine had dropped considerably and become generally affordable for Europeans.[17] Used properly, quinine could work wonders.

In the early twentieth century, many of the Europeans residing in tropical Africa took quinine on a more or less idiosyncratic basis. As the authors of the Liverpool School report on the malaria mission to Nigeria put it, "Among Europeans in West Africa, the usual practice as to the taking of quinine as a prophylactic, is to take five grains every day, or five to ten grains when they feel a little indisposed, 'out of sorts,' or when they think about it."[18] Even with irregular dosages, however, there can be little

---

[15] H. E. Annett, J. Everett Dutton, and J. H. Elliott, *Report of the Malaria Expedition to Nigeria of the Liverpool School of Tropical Medicine and Medical Parasitology. Part I: Malarial Fever, Etc. Memoir III, Liverpool School of Tropical Medicine* (Liverpool: Liverpool University Press, 1901), 48–49. See also J. Everett Dutton, *Report of the Malaria Expedition to the Gambia (1902). Memoire X* (London: Longmans, Green & Co. for the University Press of Liverpool, 1903), 33.

    The epidemiological vulnerability of Europeans in tropical Africa may also have been influenced by the social culture of African societies in whose midst they lived. In tropical African societies, there was no tradition of the intimate personal servant, as, for example, in British India. There, many Europeans had in attendance personal servants who operated a sail-like cloth fan known as a punkah. Ronald Ross held that this pattern of punkah usage constituted one of the principal epidemiological differences between the malaria risks in India and tropical Africa. [William MacGregor, Ronald Ross, J. M. Young, C. F. Fearnside, George A. Williamson, George G. Low, Rubert Wm. Boyce, Edward Henderson, Patrick Manson, J. L. Poynder, and James Cantlie, "A Discussion on Malaria and Its Prevention," *British Medical Journal*, vol. 2, no. 2124 (Sept. 14, 1901), 683.]

[16] In 1820, two French chemists isolated the two major antimalarial alkaloids, quinine and cinchonine, from the bark of the cinchona tree. For nearly two centuries before this feat, cinchona bark had been used to cure malaria, although, because the percentage of antimalarial alkaloids in cinchona bark varied greatly among the subspecies of cinchona and even from tree to tree, the effectiveness of treatment with the bark was uneven. With the rise of early chemical companies, quinine sulfate became the preferred antimalarial medication. [Webb, *Humanity's Burden*, 95–110.]

[17] The price of quinine dropped considerably in the late 1880s. See Webb, *Humanity's Burden*, 112–114.

[18] Annett, Dutton, and Elliott, *Report of the Malaria Expedition to Nigeria*, 47–48. The report's authors were skeptical of the regular use of quinine.

doubt that those who self-medicated with quinine reduced the severity of malarial infections and reduced their risk of serious complications and death.[19] Quinine usage, however, also had a darker side. For some Europeans, it could produce a deadly syndrome known as *blackwater fever*, characterized by the passage of blood in the urine.[20] (The cause of the syndrome is unknown, but it is thought to be possibly the result of an autoimmune reaction.)

Quinine in the bloodstream could not kill the sporozoite form of the malaria parasite that the mosquito injected while taking her blood meal, and it could not kill the forms of the parasite that developed soon thereafter in the liver. Quinine could, however, kill the parasites when they emerged from the liver; thus, in theory, it could interrupt the disease process, killing the parasites before they infected the hemoglobin cells. In practice, because many found that regular quinine therapy had unpleasant side effects, including nausea, strict compliance with a "prophylactic" regimen of quinine use was not the norm. Its principal virtue, among the small number of Europeans who were long-term residents in tropical Africa and who had survived the initial challenges from falciparum malaria, may have been to provide palliative relief by reducing the parasite load and thereby the disease symptoms. In this sense, for the European "old coasters," quinine worked to the same result as did many of the African plant-based medicines used to treat malaria.

Early in the twentieth century, the potential benefits of quinine use were deemed so great – and the costs of malaria so high – that military and civil authorities began to promote its broad use among Europeans. In 1906, for

[19] On late nineteenth-century quinine treatments in West Africa for malarial fever, see W. H. Crosse, *Notes on the Malarial Fevers Met with on the River Niger (West Africa)* (London: Simpkin, Marshall, Hamilton, Kent and H. H. G. Gratton, 1892), 38.
   Some Europeans with extensive experience in tropical Africa, having survived the initial challenge of falciparum malaria, eschewed the use of quinine as a prophylactic. The missionary David Livingstone, for example, judged that prophylactic quinine was of little use and held that the best protection against serious bouts of malaria was to be well housed, well clothed, and well fed. [David Livingstone, *Narrative of an Expedition to The Zambesi and Its Tributaries* (Torrington, WY: Narrative Press, 2004), 31–33.]
[20] Malariologists produced an impressive volume of research on blackwater fever in the period before 1950. Blackwater fever was diagnosed throughout the malarious world. The earliest research on blackwater fever in tropical Africa is C. W. Daniels, "Notes on 'Blackwater Fever' in British Central Africa," in *Reports to the Malaria Committee of the Royal Society*, fifth series (London: Harrison and Sons, 1901), 44–79.
   Blackwater fever largely disappeared as a diagnostic category of disease in the period after the Second World War, when chloroquine and other synthetic antimalarial drugs largely displaced quinine as the therapy of choice in cases of severe malaria.

example, the French military authorities allocated the drug even to the rank and file. After struggling with an outbreak of yellow fever and the annual onslaught of malaria, medical authorities in Dakar decided to provide French naval troops stationed in Dakar with 300 mg of quinine per day or 500 mg every second day.[21] Also in 1906, the École de Médecine tropicale in Brussels launched a public health propaganda campaign to encourage the regular use of quinine prophylaxis in the colonies, and it was supported strongly by the cohort of Italian physicians serving in the Belgian Congo.[22]

Even with quinine and mosquito netting, the risks to the European colonizers who resided in tropical Africa were great. The most fearsome region was West Africa. Newly arrived Europeans were immunologically naïve and could be swept away by deadly fever in a matter of days. Government posts were left vacant. The disease environment ate away at the political foundations the colonizers sought to establish, and in many areas of tropical Africa it ruled out any permanent European settlements.

THE DISCOVERY OF ACQUIRED IMMUNITY

In the late 1890s, the German bacteriologist Robert Koch was called to the German colony in New Guinea known as Kaiser-Wilhelms-Land to investigate a devastating epidemic of malaria among imported Chinese laborers. Through mass blood screenings of the indigenous inhabitants, Koch discovered that many adults had no clinical symptoms of malaria even though there were parasites in their blood. He began to develop an insight that laid the groundwork for the scientific appreciation of acquired immunity. Koch came to the understanding that adults who were exposed to falciparum malaria developed a tolerance to it – an acquired immunity from disease symptoms.

For Koch, this insight had important policy implications. Parasitized individuals who were asymptomatic would be effective carriers of the parasites, and, if untreated, they would participate in the ongoing transmission of the disease. This suggested to Koch that it might be possible to treat entire populations with quinine and thereby eliminate the parasites from their

---

[21] They also distributed coffee (considered to be a healthful drink) and issued the men one-half kilogram of ice per day. [Bellet, "État sanitaire de Dakar et du personnel de la Marine pendant l'hivernage de 1906," *Archives de médecine navale*, vol. 87 (1907), 424–425.]

[22] A. Duren, "Un essai d'étude d'ensemble du paludisme au Congo Belge," *Institut Royal Colonial Belge, Section des sciences naturelles et médicales. Mémoires*, vol. 5, no. 5 (1937), 62. Adults took 400–500 mg of quinine per day.

human reservoir. He tried out this program on imported Chinese laborers in a plantation setting in Kaiser-Wilhelms-Land with success.[23]

Koch launched a similar program in the port of Dar es Salaam on the eastern African coast with hopes of eliminating malaria locally and making the new colony of German East Africa safe for German occupation. It proved impossible to accomplish. He did not have the full support of the chief German medical officer in Dar es Salaam or the African populations, and the intermittent flow of migrants between the settlement of Dar es Salaam and the surrounding region likewise militated against successful implementation of the treatment scheme.[24]

The discovery of a broadly shared acquired immunity and a vast population of asymptomatic carriers called for a new approach to malaria control. It was now clear that Europeans did not principally contract malaria from one another. Another approach was badly needed.

EARLY EXPERIENCES WITH MOSQUITO CONTROL

The late-nineteenth-century discovery that anopheline mosquitoes transmitted malaria – like the discovery of acquired immunity – initially suggested revolutionary prospects for controlling malaria in tropical Africa. The hope was that the deadliest impediment to European colonization might be largely obviated. Scientists rushed to the British territories in tropical Africa to determine the feasibility and the best means to interrupt malaria transmission. In early 1899, two of the leading malaria researchers in British India, S. R. Christophers and J. W. W. Stephens, traveled to the British Central Africa Protectorate (Nyasaland/Malawi) to investigate malaria and the horrifying illness known as blackwater fever that seemed to be a complication of it. They intended to set up research facilities in Blantyre, but left after determining that the hospital and other available facilities were inadequate. C. W. Daniels of the London School of Tropical Medicine also traveled to Blantyre and stayed to conduct research on blackwater fever.[25]

---

[23] W. U. Eckart, "Malaria and Colonialism in the German Colonies New Guinea and the Cameroons. Research, Control, Thoughts of Eradication," *Parassitologia*, vol. 40 (1998), 83–90.

[24] Ann Beck, "Medicine and Society in Tanganyika, 1890–1930: A Historical Inquiry," *Transactions of the American Philosophical Society*, vol. 67, pt. 3 (1977), 14–15.

[25] Michael Gelfand, *Lakeside Pioneers: Socio-medical Study of Nyasaland (1875–1920)* (Oxford: Basil Blackwell, 1964), 251–252; C. W. Daniels, "Notes on 'Blackwater Fever' in British Central Africa," 44–79.

Most of the early British malaria investigations, however, focused on the West African coastal towns in which the British had long-standing commercial and missionary interests and where malaria had long exacted a high toll. Ronald Ross – discoverer of the anopheline vector of avian malaria and a member of the newly formed Liverpool School of Tropical Diseases – traveled with a few scientific colleagues to Freetown, Sierra Leone, in 1899.[26] Ross discovered that the chief breeding places for anophelines were puddles. The governor's health officer was unenthusiastic: he sent out one man to oil puddles to kill mosquito larvae.[27]

In 1900, the Royal Society sent an expert mission to West Africa. Christophers and Stephens headed the team. They were strongly invested in the idea of quinine prophylaxis and doubted the practicality of Ross's ideas about mosquito control. In the agglomeration of villages that constituted the town of Accra, they estimated that each village had a total of thirty to forty pits from which soil was dug for building material or for collecting rainwater and that most of the pits were suitable for anopheline breeding.[28] Variation, however, was the rule. Some sections of Accra were virtually free from *Anopheles*, others heavily infested. In their judgment, ridding whole towns of anophelines would involve many years of work to improve surface drainage.

Christophers and Stephens visited the island of Lagos and found that the situation there was extreme. Lagos was saturated by a plethora of minor lagoons. Around the lagoon margins were waterlogged lands, partially reclaimed through the deposition of mud, shell banks, and refuse. Everywhere were "innumerable pools and puddles," a seemingly limitless breeding ground for anophelines.[29] They came to the judgment that the best option to protect Europeans in West Africa was residential segregation.[30]

---

[26] Ronald Ross would be awarded the Nobel Prize in Medicine in 1902 for his malaria research.

[27] Gordon Harrison, *Mosquitoes, Malaria & Man: A History of the Hostilities Since 1880* (New York: E. P. Dutton, 1978), 123–128.

[28] S. R. Christophers and J. W. W. Stephens, "The Native as the Prime Agent in the Malarial Infection of the Europeans," in *Further Reports to the Malaria Committee of the Royal Society* (London: Harrison and Sons, 1900), 4.

[29] J. W. W. Stephens and S. R. Christophers, "On the Destruction of *Anopheles* in Lagos," in *Reports to the Malarial Committee of the Royal Society*, third series (London: Harrison and Sons, 1900), 16.

[30] S. R. Christophers and J. W. W. Stephens, "The Segregation of Europeans," in *Reports to the Malaria Committee of the Royal Society*, third series (London: Harrison and Sons, 1900), 21–24.

Also in 1900, the Liverpool School sent a malaria mission to Nigeria. It arrived in Old Calabar, an eastern coastal trading town on the Cross River. The town had been a center for British merchants during the era of the slave trades, and, in the early twentieth century, it was home to about 120 Europeans who worked either for the British colonial government or the Niger Company that traded in palm oils and other agricultural goods. The team spent five weeks investigating the malarial environment there and in Duketown, the "native town" across the creek from Old Calabar.

They discovered breeding places for the *Anopheles* mosquitoes in the numerous dugout canoes that rested along the banks of the creeks, as well as in small puddles and poorly constructed drains near the European bungalows. They noticed that the construction of roads and footpaths had thrown up new microsites for anopheline breeding.[31] The researchers also found evidence in offices that were occupied only during daylight hours that some anopheline mosquitoes took their blood meals there during the day.[32]

Echoing the views of Christophers and Stephens, the Liverpool research team judged that the best option to protect Europeans was residential segregation. The alternatives could be ruled out: it was impossible to destroy the mosquito populations, and it was impossible to administer wholesale doses of quinine to the local populations.[33]

Ross returned to Freetown in 1901, with a broader program of mosquito control in mind: the populations of all mosquitoes, not just anophelines, should be reduced as much as possible in towns and their suburbs. This would bring about a steep decline in the incidence of yellow fever, transmitted by *Aedes aegypti* mosquitoes (considered at the time to belong to the *Culex*, rather than the *Aedes*, genus), as well as malaria.[34] The yellow fever vector was highly domesticated and bred in household containers. Mosquito control thus involved a large program of garbage collection to get rid of all discarded containers that might shelter mosquito larvae.

The initial results were highly encouraging. Good strides were made, but the job never got finished. In Freetown, some thirty-two African workers were organized into a "Culex gang," to pick up garbage, and an "Anopheles gang," to destroy the vector breeding pools; progress was

---

[31] Annett, Dutton, and Elliott, *Report of the Malaria Expedition to Nigeria*, 32.

[32] Annett, Dutton, and Elliott, *Report of the Malaria Expedition to Nigeria*, 36.

[33] Annett, Dutton and Elliott, *Report of the Malaria Expedition to Nigeria*, 54.

[34] R. Ross, *First Progress Report of the Campaign Against Mosquitoes in Sierra Leone (1901)*. Memoir V, Part I. (London: University Press of Liverpool, 1901), 12–13.

"fairly rapid." Ross reported that he had not gotten a mosquito bite after the first week's antilarval work, and Lieutenant McKendrick informed Ross that he was not aware of having been bitten by a mosquito during his month's stay in Freetown.[35] The early enthusiasms were dampened by the appreciation that, to be efficacious, the antilarval measures had to be carried forward in a routine manner. Freetown received about 160 inches of rain each year, and new puddles formed in a matter of hours.

THE LOGIC OF RESIDENTIAL SEGREGATION

Christophers and Stephens, the advocates for quinine prophylaxis, argued that heavily parasitized African children and asymptomatic adults – rather than mosquitoes – represented the greatest danger to Europeans. In their view, the isolation of the European sick was futile as long as Europeans and Africans continued to live in close proximity. The infections would continue to be transmitted. They held that the obvious solution was to have Europeans live a minimum of one-half mile apart from Africans.[36] A policy of residential segregation would serve the cause of public health.[37]

The epidemiological principles proved difficult to implement. In some towns, the groundswell of race-and-health logic broke on the shoals of everyday practice. African schoolchildren were often resident on the grounds of the European-run Christian missions.[38] European business and government interests were enmeshed with those of local communities.

[35] Ross, *First Progress Report*, 6–7, 9.
[36] S. R. Christophers and J. W. W. Stephens, "The Segregation of Europeans," 23; S. R. Christophers and J. W. W. Stephens, "The Native as the Prime Agent in the Malarial Infection of Europeans," 16–18.
    In 1901, they reiterated the case for residential segregation, drawing on their nearly two years' experiences in African towns including Blantyre, Accra, and Freetown and in the African bush: *Anopheles* flew, at most, a few hundred yards from their breeding sites. [J. W. W. Stephens and S. R. Christophers, "The Proposed Site for European Residences in the Freetown Hill," in *Reports to the Malaria Committee of the Royal Society*, fifth series (London, 1901), 5.]
[37] The application of the principle could be extended to work settings beyond the towns. Stephens and Christophers proposed a graduated schema. During the construction of rail lines, for example, European temporary residences should be sited one mile from the nearest African village. The African laborers should be camped at a minimum of one-half mile from the Europeans, and the house servants should sleep at least one-quarter mile from the European compounds. Only one personal servant should be allowed to remain near the European quarters at night. [J. W. W. Stephens and S. R. Christophers, "Note on Malarial Fever Contracted on Railways (under Construction)," in *Reports to the Malarial Committee of the Royal Society*, third series (London, 1900), 21.]
[38] Daniels, "Prophylaxis," 43.

Interracial or closely adjoining racial neighborhoods were often the rule –
for example, in Bathurst in the Gambia, Conakry in French Guinea, and
Lagos in Southern Nigeria.

For this reason, some colonial administrators explicitly rejected residential segregation to control malaria. Sir William MacGregor, the British
Governor of Southern Nigeria, made his argument on both practical and
moral grounds:

> It is strongly recommended in certain competent quarters that to get away from
> infected mosquitos [sic] Europeans should live at places apart from the natives. This
> may be called the academic view. From the administrative point of view it is an
> unacceptable doctrine. The academic view is ungenerous, and would afford no
> radical remedy were it practicable, which it is not. The policy followed in Lagos in
> this as in other matters is to take the native along with the European on the way
> leading to improvement. Here they cannot live apart nor work apart, and they
> should not try to do so. Separation would mean that little, or at least less, would be
> done for the native, and the admitted source of infection would remain perennial.
> To simply protect the European from fever here would never make Lagos the great
> commercial port that it should become. What we can do in this matter for the
> uneducated part of the Lagos population will be effected chiefly by reclaiming the
> swamps and administering quinine.[39]

Both government and private organizations were enlisted in the struggle to
reduce the impact of urban malaria. In 1901, Governor MacGregor introduced the ninety-five members of the Lagos Ladies' League, with an
entirely African membership, to Ronald Ross, who professed that they
would succeed in doing very much good by preaching "the use of quinine,
the prevention of fever by scientific methods, and the cleanliness of private
houses."[40]

In some West African colonies, however, the racial segregation paradigm had considerable purchase, and it justified a variety of initiatives. In
Sierra Leone, the colonial government established a European residential
compound atop a hill on the outskirts of Freetown, with a railway link to

---

[39] MacGregor et al., "A Discussion on Malaria and Its Prevention," 682.

 MacGregor also noted that mosquitoes were "much more numerous" around the
European quarters than the native dwellings, and he attributed this to the larger number
of tanks, pools, and other water receptacles of the Europeans. The more numerous
mosquitoes that he observed may well have been culicines, rather than anophelines; the
Liverpool expedition to the Cross River region, however, had noted that anophelines bred
in the cups of water that protected from ants the wooden piles supporting European
bungalows. [MacGregor et al., "A Discussion on Malaria and Its Prevention," 682;
Annett et al., Report of the Malaria Expedition, 8–9.]

[40] [Anon.], "The Antimalaria Campaign. The Liverpool Malaria Expedition," British
Medical Journal, vol. 2 (7 September 1901), 644.

the town. In the Gold Coast, the colonial government demolished "slum" housing in Accra and Sekondi and laid plans to establish separate residential spaces for Africans and Europeans. All was done in the name of malaria prevention.[41]

EARLY ADVANCES IN EPIDEMIOLOGY

The early prospects for success in malaria control opened up new vistas in epidemiology and clinical treatment. C. W. Daniels stressed the need to determine the extent of malarial infections in Freetown in order to prioritize interventions and determine their efficacy. Daniels recommended a study to estimate the splenic enlargement of the children of Freetown in different age groups and an examination of the Barbadians in the West Indian regiment who had not previously been exposed to malaria, along with their length of residency in Sierra Leone, as a proxy check for the vulnerability of nonimmune Europeans.[42]

In 1904, a new procedure using Giemsa stain made the parasites in the blood slides more easily visible under the microscope. This gave investigators the means to measure the percentages of a sampled population that had one or more species of malaria parasites in their bloodstreams, known as the *parasite rates*. The technique of palpating the spleen became widely known and practiced, and this allowed for the collection of data on the percentages of the population with different degrees of splenic distention, known as the *spleen rates*.[43] These techniques threw new light on the extent of malaria parasitization in tropical Africa.

These techniques, however, had significant limitations. Thin blood smears gave lower readings of parasite density than did semi-thick or thick smears. The more time that one spent looking for parasites, the more one found; thus, parasite densities were in part a function of the expertise of the

---

[41] Raymond E. Dumett, "The Campaign against Malaria and the Expansion of Scientific Medical and Sanitary Services in British West Africa, 1898–1910," *African Historical Studies*, vol. 1, no. 2 (1968), 170.

[42] Appendix. Letter from C. W. Daniels to Ronald Ross, 1 October 1901, in R. Ross, *First Progress Report of the Campaign Against Mosquitoes in Sierra Leone (1901)*, 21–22. On the career of C. W. Daniels, see G. C. Cook, "Charles Wilberforce Daniels, FRCP (1862–1927): Underrated Pioneer of Tropical Medicine," *Acta Tropica*, vol. 81 (2002), 237–250.

[43] Gustav Geimsa published an academic paper in 1904 that disseminated information about the stain and the technique for using. Today, it is still one of the most widely utilized laboratory procedures. [Bernhard Fleischer, "Editorial: 100 Years Ago: Giemsa's Solution for Staining of Plasmodia," *Tropical Medicine and International Health*, vol. 9, no. 7 (2004), 755–756.]

microscopist and the time devoted to each slide.[44] Moreover, the parasite rates did not correlate well with disease symptoms because some individuals with acquired immunities were asymptomatic and yet highly parasitized. Many other individuals who had acquired immunity to malaria suppressed their parasitemia to low levels, and thus the low parasite densities were often indicators of acquired immunity that, in turn, indicated high levels of transmission. The levels of gametocytes – the sexual stages of the parasite life cycle – taken from a prominent vein were not a reliable indicator of infectivity because, after their formation, the gametocytes migrated to the tiny capillaries, where a mosquito would more likely pick up the gametocytes during her blood meal. The palpation of the spleen by a skilled practitioner was highly reliable in determining the extent of childhood infections and levels of parasitemia, but with the acquisition of immunity, the distension of the spleen generally subsided, and many individuals without enlarged spleens were parasitized. For these reasons, and the fact that the numbers of parasites in the blood would wax and wane with the rigors of the cyclical fevers, early microscopy and physical examination could only partially capture the dynamics of infection and transmission.

Some research issues, however, were more or less straightforward, and, on these, the first generation of malariologists made good progress. One important question was: What was the species composition of the parasite mosaics or, as it was referred to at the time, the parasite prevalence? This question was taken up in West Africa beginning in 1912, when yellow fever investigators began to turn their attention to malaria. From the yellow fever laboratories in Accra, Sekondi, and Freetown, evidence began to accumulate that falciparum parasites (referred to as "subtertian") were predominant and thus that malarial infections in West Africa demonstrated a very different parasite mix than that found in India. In 1916, J. C. B. Stratham, in Freetown, reported that falciparum parasites constituted some 98.5 percent of the 676 cases that he studied.[45]

Over time, the collection of data on the parasitization of the non-African residents in some towns became routinized. In Dar es Salaam, for example, government and private practitioners notified the authorities

---

[44] The major three malaria plasmodia were identified in the late nineteenth century: *Plasmodium vivax* and *Plasmodium malariae* by G. B. Grassi and R. Feletti in 1890; and *Plasmodium falciparum* by W. Welsh in 1897. J. W. W. Stephens identified *Plasmodium ovale* as a parasite distinct from *Plasmodium vivax* in 1922. The early twentieth-century readings of blood slides in tropical Africa misidentified *P. ovale*, usually as *P. vivax*.
[45] J. W. S Macfie and A. Ingram, "Observations on Malaria in the Gold Coast Colony, West Africa," *Annals of Tropical Medicine and Parasitology*, vol. 11 (1918), 2–5.

of the malaria cases that they treated, and, from these notifications, maps were made that covered all of the Europeans and "a certain proportion of the Indian residents." The extent of malarial infection in the African population was done by a spleen survey of the children. These studies could then be linked to entomological surveys to determine, for example, if the creek-bred anophelines were more responsible for malarial infections than were local puddle-breeders. (This was confounded somewhat by the observation that, in Khartoum, as the town breeding sites were eliminated, mosquitoes flew in from great distances, thus necessitating the extension of antimalaria operations well beyond the town.)[46] Another technique to establish vector competence – that is, the ability of the different anopheline mosquitoes to transmit malaria – was to have the mosquitoes feed on parasitized African children who had high densities of gametocytes in their blood and later to dissect the mosquitoes for evidence of parasite infection.[47]

Those Europeans in the African tropics who were not part of the small medical and scientific communities only slowly developed an appreciation for the insights gained from malaria epidemiology. In the coastal port of Sekondi, Gold Coast (now, Ghana), the European community planned to establish a club on terrain bounded by a swamp and an African village. The construction of a railroad there went forward without any consideration for its likely impact on vector-borne disease.[48] The political needs of governance, too, could override over epidemiological concerns. Experts from the Liverpool School thought, for example, that the best approach to malaria control in Kumasi, located in the upcountry Gold Coast, would be to remove the seat of district government to a healthier locality, but this suggestion was roundly ignored.[49]

[46] A. McKenzie, "A Distribution of Malaria in Dar es Salaam," *Kenya and East African Medical Journal*, vol. 4 (1927–1928), 164–180.

[47] R. M. Gordon and G. Macdonald, "Transmission of Malaria in Sierra Leone," *Annals of Tropical Medicine and Parasitology*, vol. 24, no. 1 (1930), 75–76.

[48] Lieut.-Colonel Giles, *General Sanitation and Anti-Malarial Measures in Sekondi, The Goldfields and Kumassi* (London: Williams & Norgate for the University Press of Liverpool, 1905), 2–3. Giles noted "the engineering works in connection with the railway have, as is so often the case in the Tropics, greatly intensified the sanitary difficulties of the case. The embankment of the permanent way and the borrow-pits on its sides, now form permanent breeding places for mosquitoes; whereas, but for this, after the prolonged drought that Sekondi experienced at the time of our visit, there would have been no natural breeding places whatever on the site."

[49] Giles, *General Sanitation and Anti-Malarial Measures*, 16.

THE EARLY INSTANCES OF CONTROL-AND-LAPSE

In those same early years when Christophers and Stephens advocated for residential segregation, Ross and his colleagues, convinced of the practicality of larval control, continued their investigations. In 1901, M. Logan Taylor assayed the mosquito control prospects in Freetown (Sierra Leone), Cape Coast (Gold Coast), and Accra (Gold Coast), and he rejected outright the view than mosquito control was impracticable in West Africa. In his view, with proper methods, it would be possible to reduce the mosquito populations by at least 80 or 90 percent.[50] Taylor also made observations about the sanitary systems of both towns for the disposal of human waste. Governor MacGregor in Southern Nigeria had given the appalling figure of 42 percent infantile mortality before the age of one year and attributed the deaths to fever and "bowel complaints."[51] In 1902, Taylor surveyed the towns of Cape Coast and Sekondi and recommended the establishment of sanitary boards.[52] General sanitation soon emerged as a paradigm that was intimately linked to malaria control.

The findings of the malaria missions were surprising. Anophelines did not restrict their breeding to very shallow surface pools of water. In Bathurst, J. E. Dutton headed a Liverpool School of Tropical Medicine expedition that discovered that anophelines would breed in any collection of water, as did the culicines.[53] The chief breeding places were canoes, boats, lighters, and cutters along the shore. The expedition's analysis of fifty boats produced an estimate of two thousand mosquitoes per week per vessel.[54] And Dutton also made a discovery that turned upside down notions about general sanitation, mosquitoes, and relative wealth:

The number of mosquito breeding-places present in compounds is found to vary with the social position of the occupier. In small compounds of the poorer natives, where one or two huts were present, no breeding places were found. These natives had no discarded bottles, etc., in which water could collect, nor were wells or tubs

---

[50] M. Logan Taylor, "Sanitary Work in West Africa," *British Medical Journal*, vol. 2, no. 2177 (20 September 1902), 852–853. His report was also published as M. Logan Taylor, *Second Progress Report of the Campaign Against Mosquitoes in Sierra Leone.* Memoir V. Part 2. Liverpool School of Tropical Medicine (Liverpool: University Press of Liverpool, 1902).

[51] [Anon.], "The Antimalaria Campaign," 644.

[52] London School of Hygiene and Tropical Medicine, Ross Archives, Cabinet A, Drawer II, File 13, Dr. M. Logan Taylor, *Report on Sanitary Conditions at Cape Coast with Suggestions as to Improvement*, 23 April 1902. Cited by Dumett, "The Campaign Against Malaria," 168, note 85.

[53] Dutton, *Report of the Malaria Expedition to the Gambia 1902*, 1.

[54] Dutton, *Report of the Malaria Expedition to the Gambia, 1902*, 18.

or any article for the storage of water present, sufficient water for the day being drawn from one of the public wells. These compounds were exceedingly clean and tidy, and no mosquitoes were found breeding in them. Excepting these, breeding-places were found and increased in extent and number in proportion to the wealth and position of the occupier of the compound, reaching a maximum on the premises of the larger traders (natives and white), where innumerable facilities for the development of mosquitoes were afforded.[55]

Dutton came to the conclusion that of the three approaches to malaria control on the table – the wholesale use of quinine by Europeans, residential segregation, and mosquito control – only mosquito control was feasible. It would have the benefit of reducing the risk of yellow fever and filariasis, in addition to malaria.[56] The leaders of a mission to Conakry, where native houses were in close proximity to those of the Europeans, also expressed optimism for mosquito control.[57]

The core difficulty was that, to be successful, the colonial governments needed to pursue mosquito control unremittingly. The work was dull, repetitive, and always fell short: there were always going to be some malarial infections. Moreover, when mosquito control did succeed in reducing infections, it was difficult to ascribe success convincingly to it because the incidence of malaria tended to vary over time. For these reasons, mosquito control did not command the general respect of the European communities who stood to benefit from it, and it fared poorly among the competing demands for government monies.

This contributed to a pattern of repetitive control-and-lapse episodes. In Freetown, for example, after the initial burst of enthusiasm, the control efforts became less thorough. By the end of the first decade of the twentieth century, Freetown had become once again heavily malarious. The problem gained the attention of the Colonial Office in 1917, when, during the rainy season, troops from South Africa and New Zealand became infected with malaria while onboard their ships in the harbor at Freetown. Some troop transports arrived in England with their crews crippled and with men on board suffering from fevers, and laboratory evidence confirmed that the

---

[55] Dutton, *Report of the Malaria Expedition to the Gambia, 1902*, 25.
[56] Dutton, *Report of the Malaria Expedition to the Gambia 1902*, 34–35. Dutton recommended the adoption of the segregation principle in the construction of any new administrative housing.
[57] R. Boyce, A. Evans, and H.H. Clarke, *Report on the Sanitation and Anti-Malarial Measures in Practice in Bathurst, Conakry, and Freetown* (London: University Press of Liverpool, 1905), 20.

infections – some of which were fatal – were due to malaria.[58] Malaria control in Freetown was vigorously reengaged until July 1918, when the global influenza pandemic reached Freetown and killed more than 1,000 of its 5,000 residents. In the aftermath of the pandemic, malaria control reforms were again put in place, but after the First World War, they again lapsed.[59]

During the interwar period, this pattern was repeated in the French and British West African coastal towns in which Europeans were resident. Mosquito control efforts were episodic and reactionary, stepped up only during times of heightened sickness.[60] It seemed to be the most that could be accomplished in an era of severe financial constraints.

Elsewhere in tropical Africa and in South Africa, there were variations on the pattern. The Portuguese colonies of Angola and Mozambique had distinctive colonial histories that influenced their path of malaria control. In the major coastal towns of Angola and Mozambique, the Luso-African communities had a long-established presence that extended back to the late fifteenth and sixteenth centuries of European exploration and trade. The death rates from malaria in the coastal towns had been notoriously high among newly arrived European traders and immigrants. In the early twentieth century, Portuguese traders and physicians used quinine to treat malaria, but the Portuguese authorities did not adopt the practice of residential segregation, and they did not engage in mosquito control. Over time, however, the growth of the cities entailed public works projects that reduced anopheline habitat and contributed to a reduction in malaria transmission.

---

[58] NAUK, CO 267/579, "Report on Suggested Anti-Malarial Measures at Freetown," attached to Edward J. Steedman to Director General, Medical Department of the Navy, 16 March 1918, Sierra Leone. At some points during the war years, up to forty or fifty ships had been counted to lie in the Freetown harbor at the same time.

 The sanitary authorities in Sierra Leone had earlier tried to reject the assertion that troops had contracted malaria while on board ship in the Freetown harbor; Ronald Ross weighed in, writing "I myself saw three of the cases, and also verified the diagnosis of malaria in their blood." [NAUK. CO 267/576. War Office. "Malaria Contracted at Sierra Leone and Dakar" (n. d., 1917)].

[59] NAUK, CO267/580. R. H. Cordner, "Anti-Malarial Campaign During 1918. Military Areas." 24 December 1918.

[60] In Dakar, for example, during a bad malarial season in 1933, the Sanitary Service carried out an extensive larviciding program and filled in wells and streambeds, among other public works activities, in an effort to reduce the levels of transmission. [C. Gilly, "Activité du Service d'Hygiène de la Circonscription de Dakar pendant l'hivernage 1933 (1er juin au 1er décembre)," *Bulletin de la Société de pathologie exotique et de ses filiales*, vol. 27, no. 1 (1934), 91–93.]

In South Africa, over the course of nineteenth century, British colonists expanded their farming frontier to the east from Cape Province. Coastal ports grew up to serve the export-oriented British farmers. There, the dynamics of urban growth dramatically reduced malaria transmission: the authorities oversaw the drainage and filling-in of lowlands to make room for new buildings, and anopheline habitat disappeared. East London and Durban, for example, had been malarious in the late nineteenth century, yet as the settlements grew into cities, they became better drained, and malaria all but disappeared.[61] This anticipated a general reduction of the intensity of malaria transmission in modernizing urban environments elsewhere in Africa south of the Sahara.

MALARIA CONTROL IN THE MINING CITIES AND URBAN LOWLANDS

The most focused efforts at malaria control, however, emerged in entirely new settlements – on sites either that were nearby mineral resources or had been converted to plantations to grow export crops. In both, the emphasis was on creating environments that were safe for Europeans and that reduced African morbidity to a level that interfered little with worker productivity. Where there was no firmly established pattern of cross-cultural, Euro-African settlement, the Europeans typically chose to live apart from their African workers and thereby initiated a de facto policy of residential segregation based on race. This practice was true of the Belgians, the Germans, the British, and the French.

The earliest and most successful interventions were in Northern Rhodesia (now Zambia) near rich copper deposits. There, a combination of environmental engineering; larviciding; metal screening of windows, doors, and eaves; and the prophylactic and curative use of quinine reduced malaria to a very minor health issue. This impressive achievement was owing, in good measure, to the initiative and vision of Malcolm Watson, a malariologist who had pioneered environmental engineering in Malaya with powerful consequences for the rubber industry there and who hoped to create a model of health and economic growth that would redound to the benefit of both Europeans and Africans.[62] The mining companies were

---

[61] Comment of Fleet-Surgeon W. E. Home in J. G. Thomson, "Endemic and Epidemic Malaria in Southern Rhodesia, *Proceedings of the Royal Society of Medicine*, vol. 22, no. 8 (26 April 1929), 1058.

[62] Malcolm Watson, *African Highway: The Battle for Health in Central Africa* (London: John Murray, 1953).

willing to finance the antimalaria programs because they realized that the exploitation of the region's high-value mineral wealth required a disciplined and healthy African and European workforce. This multistranded high-impact model of malaria control was not fully replicated outside the zone of the Northern Rhodesian copper reserves, although its historical success there has continued to inspire some scholars who consider it a model intervention.[63]

Elsewhere, as in the cities along the copper reserves in the eastern Congo, malaria interventions took place with generally good results. Ironically, the reduction in malaria transmission meant that it was difficult to achieve fuller compliance with prescribed antimalarial practices. At least some Europeans who had survived the initial potentially deadly malarial challenges, often with curative quinine treatment, judged that running the risk of getting malaria was more attractive than taking quinine prophylaxis. In the 1920s, for example, in the mining town of Elisabethville (now Lubumbashi) in the Katanga province of the Belgian Congo, both the colonial state and the mining companies dispensed free quinine and mosquito nets to their European employees. According to a 1931 survey, 84 percent of the European population took quinine prophylactically, 10 percent took it irregularly, and 6 percent took never took quinine prophylactically. Nearly a third of the survey respondents reported having had malaria, but the percentages were lower among the group that took quinine regularly. Despite best efforts to protect the Europeans, malaria remained a problem.[64]

Residential segregation itself, as an antimalaria measure, could be quite haphazard. Most colonial planners and administrators paid scant attention to mosquito breeding sites and flight ranges. Residential segregation was at least as important in defining the racial identity of the European colonizers as it was in protecting Europeans from malarial infection. In the Belgian Congo, many European neighborhoods in the burgeoning cities were "protected" from African neighborhoods by a barrier of between 250 and 500 meters planted with rows of trees to "screen" the anopheline mosquitoes and reduce European infections. Belgian public health officials

[63] J. Utzinger, Y. Tozan, F. Doumani, and B. H. Singer, "The Economic Payoffs of Integrated Malaria Control in the Zambian Copperbelt between 1930 and 1950," *Tropical Medicine and International Health*, vol. 7, no. 8 (2002), 657–677.

[64] More than 80 percent of the respondents slept under mosquito nets – and this usage was highly correlated with regular quinine prophylaxis. U. Colombo, "Prophylaxie individuelle antimalarienne parmi la population européenne d'Elisabethville (Katanga)," *Annales de la Société belge de médecine tropicale*, vol. 11, no. 4 (1931), 373–385.

tried to impose measures to ensure that the European populations protected their houses from mosquito invasion. As early as 1913, legislation required all European houses in the Belgian Congo to be outfitted with metal screens on all windows and doors that opened to the outdoors. In practice, most European houses – even those in isolated areas – came into compliance by the late 1930s, and, by this time, most Europeans had adopted the use of the bed net.[65]

The urban settlements in lowland areas were problematic owing to their proximity to mosquito breeding grounds. Here, public works projects could make a large difference in malaria transmission. The Belgians undertook extensive drainage works in the Congo, channeling away water from swamps in Boma, Matadi, Léopoldville, Coquilhatville, and Elisabethville. They drained waters from the European residential blocs, the African *cités*, and from the industrial and commercial centers. The goals of these public works projects, however, were to extend the water, sewage, and road systems and create urban sites suitable for new construction. The dramatic reductions in malarial infections were for the most part a fortuitous boon. By the late 1930s, in the depths of the global economic depression, these public works investments were restricted to the largest urban areas. They benefited roughly one-third of the European population in the Belgian Congo and 100,000 Africans who lived in the sprawl surrounding the Europeanized urban cores.[66]

The public works projects, however, not infrequently created new mosquito breeding habitats at the same time that they reduced overall transmission. New buildings, roads, and railroads meant digging up the soil, which left behind furrows, pits, and other depressions in which mosquitoes might breed. Town growth could reduce the incidence of malarial infections, but the process was far from linear. Urban growth governed intelligently could reduce malaria. Urban sprawl, by contrast, could have epidemiologically dangerous consequences.

In Kenya, the coastal island of Mombasa was the site of an engineering effort to control malaria during the first decades of British rule. The local environment initially seemed to conspire against mosquito control. A low-lying rice swamp was a notorious breeding ground, and a quarter-mile long cutting had to be dug deep to drain it. The cut had to be made in sandy soil, however, and, with heavy showers, the sides collapsed. The local quarry was used to absorb water drained from the swamps, but the

---

[65] Duren, "Un essai d'étude d'ensemble du paludisme au Congo Belge," 59–60.
[66] Duren, "Un essai d'étude d'ensemble du paludisme au Congo Belge," 56–57.

transported silt sealed the quarry bottom and rendered it no longer porous. The result was that the quarry itself had to be oiled to prevent mosquito breeding. By 1926, however, the antimalarial efforts began to pay off, and, by 1928, H. S. de Boer thought that most cases on the island were imported. Anophelines themselves were rare.[67]

MALARIA INTERVENTIONS IN THE URBAN HIGHLANDS

Many highland areas were above an altitude of malaria transmission. In the early years of colonial occupation and settlement, the near-absence of malaria in the eastern African highlands led European settlers to a general neglect of preventative measures. In colonial Kenya, for example, highland settlers initially did not regard malaria as a serious health threat.

Their views changed dramatically during the epidemics of the 1920s.[68] In 1926, a highland epidemic broke out in Kisumu, a town on the shores of Lake Victoria. Exceptionally high rainfall had broken down a series of dams and created a large swamp that extended to within one mile of the town.[69] Mosquito densities soared, and infections followed. That same year, in Nairobi, a malarial outbreak unexpectedly ripped through the European population. It provoked a wholesale change in attitude toward mosquito control in the highland towns, and oiling and draining measures were put into place.[70] The medical authorities sought to emulate an Italian model, eliminating anophelines in the urban settlement and an area stretching three kilometers beyond. The principal requirements for success, as ever, were unrelenting diligence and nearly continuous monitoring. If a once-controlled area were to be reinvaded, the work of years could be undone in a few months.[71] And it was essential to know just which anopheline mosquitoes one was going to war against. As H. S. de Boer, who prepared a paper on malaria control for the Kenyan Branch of the British Medical Association, noted, the correct

---

[67] H. S. de Boer, "Malaria and Its Control on Mombasa Island," *Kenya and East African Medical Journal*, vol. 5, no. 1 (1928), 2–11.

[68] See, for example, J. McP. Campbell, "Malaria in the Uasin Gishu and Trans Nzoia," *Kenya and East African Medical Journal*, vol. 6, no. 2 (1929), 32–43.

[69] C. B. Symes, "Notes on Anophelines and Malaria in Kenya," *Kenya and East African Medical Journal*, vol. 5, no. 5 (1928), 176.

[70] Symes, "Notes on Anophelines and Malaria in Kenya," 157–158.

[71] H. S. de Boer, "Anti Malarial Measures in Towns," *Kenya and East African Medical Journal*, vol. 7, no. 9 (1930), 265.

answer to the question "'When is a malaria survey necessary?'" was "always."[72]

In 1928, warm and wet weather conspired to yield a bumper crop of anophelines in the Lumbwa Reserve in the highlands of Kenya. Malaria broke out. Imported, parasitized Kavirondo (Masaai) laborers who had come to work on the European farms accelerated it into an epidemic. At its peak, the European farmers found their laborers sickened – between 30 and 50 percent were too ill to work, and the number of dead in the Lumbwa Reserve went uncounted. The colonial authorities improvised, setting up local dispensaries to treat the ill and mixing quinine into whisky bottles filled with water, with instructions to local men to return to their communities and give two tablespoons of the mixture to stricken adults and smaller doses to children. Some 57,600 doses of 10 grains of quinine were thus distributed.[73]

The highland epidemics in Kenya focused imperial attention on the issue of African malaria. On Armistice Day 1928, in Nairobi, the Prince of Wales offered his view that an antimalaria campaign in Kenya would produce a hundred-fold acceleration of progress.[74] Toward this end, experts from other regions of the British Empire visited the colony to give their advice. S. P. James, a prominent malariologist who had worked extensively in India, recommended the creation of a new organization to be named The Malaria Survey of Kenya, following the British colonial model in India.[75] The Medical Department declared a new policy to liberate Kenyan towns "from the menace of malaria once and for all," and James recommended malaria be made a notifiable disease in Nairobi and that a special medical officer in Nairobi look after all antimosquito measures.[76] H. Leigh Bennett, the executive engineer in the Federated Malay States, visited the Kenyan highlands and gave advice on antimalarial drainage, including the planting of eucalyptus trees to dry out the swamps.[77]

[72] de Boer, "Anti Malarial Measures in Towns," 263, citing with approval a bulletin of the Indian malaria service.
[73] J. H. H. Chataway, "Report on the Malaria Epidemic in the Lumbwa Reserve," *Kenya and East African Medical Journal*, vol. 5 (1928–1929), 303–309.
[74] S. P. James, *Report on a Visit to Kenya and Uganda to Advise on Antimalarial Measures* (London: Crown Agents for the Colonies, 1929), 5.
[75] James, *Report on a Visit to Kenya and Uganda*, 8–16.
[76] James, *Report on a Visit to Kenya and Uganda*, 16–19.
[77] H. Leigh Bennett, "Anti-Malarial Drainage," *Kenya and East African Medical Journal*, vol. 7, no. 7 (1930), 190–198.

When sufficient resources could be allocated, the results were strongly positive. Malaria was estimated to be responsible for about 5 percent of all deaths in Nairobi over the period 1925–1938, but, by 1940, the incidence of malaria had dropped considerably. This was due in part to the fact that modern, piped water supplies served "practically the whole area." Moreover, the main roads were surfaced with tar, asphalt, or lateritic soil. Yet, as ever, there was more to be done: the anophelines continued to breed in areas overgrown in long grass and scrub plants within the municipal area.[78]

THE EARLY IMPACTS OF URBAN MALARIA CONTROL

In the years before 1945, malaria control in tropical Africa involved experimentation with mosquito "source reduction" through the destruction of mosquito habitat through drainage, or by oiling, larviciding with copper arsenate ("Paris Green"), and public works projects. In some colonies, it also involved the distribution of quinine and bed nets to Europeans to protect them against malaria; these efforts were concentrated in urban areas. The success was considerable: a lower level of malaria transmission and a consequent reduction in malaria deaths and severe illness. Over time, the urban areas became centers of starkly lower transmission than rural areas, and some of the Africans, as well as the Europeans, who were stricken with malaria in urban areas had access to quinine treatment.

Large-scale environmental engineering worked in environments in which controlled drainage was feasible, yet it was deemed too expensive to carry out in most colonial settings. Only when special conditions obtained – where there was a substantial stream of revenue and a sizeable, resident European population – could large projects be practical. These conditions were spectacularly met in the mining areas of Central Africa. In the "Copperbelt" of Northern Rhodesia and in the Katanga province of the Belgian Congo, for example, the enclave economies produced sufficient wealth that private mining companies found that it made good sense to drain the low-lying wetlands to destroy mosquito habitat. This foundation was further improved through the screening of residential housing and chemical treatment of the sick. These programs produced a significant improvement in the health of African workers, reducing labor days lost to disease and, at the same time, dramatically decreasing the mortal risk to

---

[78] C. B. Symes, "Malaria in Nairobi," *East African Medical Journal*, vol. 17 (1940), 298, 302.

European mining specialists and their families.[79] A substantial risk was, however, passed on to the children of the African mine workers, who grew up as nonimmunes. They faced severe illness or even death when taken on visits to the rural villages in which other family members lived. Full protection could lead to fatal vulnerability.

Intermittent malaria control could produce vulnerabilities at the population level as well, when transmission was reduced so low that urban African communities lost their acquired immunities. During the Second World War, the port of Freetown was of critical importance to the Allied war effort, and mosquito control there was prosecuted vigorously. The incidence of clinical malaria among the troops in the military services and in shipping was sharply reduced. This success was accompanied, however, by an increase in the severity of malarial infections in older age cohorts in the African populations. The Malaria Control Unit in Freetown signaled this disturbing discovery in 1944 and raised a red flag. The concern was that future lapses in mosquito control might produce epidemic malaria among the African populations:

The information obtained by examination of the African population also shows a marked diminution in the incidence of infection but with the consequent loss in immunity and shift to higher age groups the clinical signs accompanying an infection have become more marked. If control is maintained at its present level for the next two or three years then lapses both Freetown and Kissy will run the risk of epidemic malaria with its high mortality.[80]

A year later, the Malaria Control Unit judged that malaria control had reduced the parasite rate in the African population to the lowest figures considered possible and confirmed that this success had been accompanied by the increased severity of malarial infections in the African population.[81] On this basis, requests were made for monies to continue malaria control in Freetown after the conclusion of the war. The requests went unfunded. Malaria was resurgent in Freetown, but the consequences of epidemic malaria went unstudied.

The problematic of European vulnerability – how to protect nonimmunes by preventing malaria transmission to the greatest extent feasible and by

---

[79] Watson, *African Highway*; Utzinger et al., "The Economic Payoffs of Integrated Malaria Control in the Zambian Copperbelt," 657–677.

[80] NAUK, CO 554/137/5. Malaria Control Unit. Quarterly Report: July-Sept. [1944; Freetown, Sierra Leone], 14.

[81] NAUK, CO544/137/6. G. A. Walton, "Quarterly Progress Report, Malaria Control Unit, Freetown, Third Quarter 1945," 19.

treating infections with quinine – was at the forefront of control efforts. The problematic of African partial immunity – how to prevent malaria transmission to the greatest extent feasible and how to prevent epidemic malaria among communities who had lost their acquired immunities – was not of pressing concern to the policy-makers and government officials who controlled the purse strings.

2

African Immunity

As the families of European administrators, military officers, traders, plantation owners, mining specialists, and missionaries struggled with their own vulnerabilities to malaria, the European medical community and the new specialists in malariology grappled with the seeming differences between the health of the Europeans in the African tropics and the Africans in whose midst they lived. Over the course of the first several decades of the twentieth century, the idea that Africans did not suffer from malaria dissipated, but a sense of profound difference remained. The fact that virtually all Africans were or had been at one time infected with malaria parasites led most in the biomedical community to the view that the partial or even full immunity of African adults was a condition that generally did not require therapeutic interventions. Some held that curative antimalarial treatment for adult Africans could be dangerous because it might jeopardize their acquired immunity to malaria.

The issue of the burden of malaria for African children was fraught with contradictions and remained highly contested into the immediate post-Second World War period. Some specialists held that there was little childhood mortality that could be attributed to malarial infections. Others believed that malaria was a major killer of children.

AFRICAN STRATEGIES AGAINST MOSQUITOES

Tropical Africans had suffered the heavy burden of malaria and other vector-borne infectious diseases for many millennia. Although the inhabitants of most African communities, like most communities throughout the wider world, did not understand that mosquito bites could cause human disease, they nonetheless had devised ingenious methods to reduce the annoyance of buzzing and biting mosquitoes, particularly during the evenings and nights when the insects prevented sound sleep.

One of the most effective ways to reduce mosquito annoyance was to set a smoky fire. This worked well as an evening repellent for those who could situate themselves within the drifting plumes of the smoke drafts inside a hut.[1] Another approach was to apply ointments made from plants with aromas that repelled the mosquitoes; sometimes the plant leaves were dipped in gasoline or lamp oil to enhance their powers. Yet another approach was to craft mosquito traps from plant leaves dipped in watery fermented maize powder that attracted mosquitoes, which then got stuck to the leaves.

In sleeping quarters, where the free movement of air was restricted, the principal strategy, however, apart from swatting mosquitoes, was to fumigate. The challenge was to produce enough acrid smoke to debilitate or drive away the mosquitoes, but not so much as to make breathing difficult. Fumigation caused eye and respiratory system irritations and infections. Most deemed these occasional problems an acceptable cost to pay for a generally better night's sleep.

Africans used a broad array of plants for fumigation. Two of the most widely employed in western Africa were the oil palm tree (*Eleais guineensis*) and the coconut palm tree (*Cocos nucifera*). The male flower of the oil palm, placed on the embers of a fire, produced an acrid smoke that stunned or killed mosquitoes outright. Other parts of the oil palm were similarly put to use. The fibers of palm pulp that had been pressed for oil burned nicely when rolled up in balls or pressed into disks, as did the husks of the palm kernels. Even fibers from the trunks of old oil palm trees that had been felled could serve the same purpose. The fibers of coconuts and other parts of the coconut palm tree were also prized as antimosquito fumigants.[2]

---

[1] On the native reserves in colonial Kenya, the entomologist C. B. Symes noted:

> The greater numbers of mosquitoes found in native huts without fires than in huts with fires is a constant observation. In the lake-shore villages there are huts set apart for unmarried boys and girls, in which no cooking is done and no fires are made. The occupants of these huts take their meals in the huts of the elder married members, where fires are almost continuously burning. Babies remain with their mothers until they reach the age of about five or six years when they sleep in the fireless huts with the other youths and unmarried members of the village. The protection afforded by the smoke of fires therefore is not available for any children after they leave their mothers' huts. [Symes, "Notes on Anophelines and Malaria in Kenya," 181.]

[2] In Senegal and the Gambia, tree kernels principally from the tree *Daniella oliveri* were mixed with perfumed resins and burned in pots. The smoke from these *churai* mixtures did

Another approach to mosquito control was to position a physical barrier to protect the sleeper from the flying insects. Along the coastline of Dahomey (now Benin) in the nineteenth century (and probably much earlier), African communities fashioned mosquito nets both from cotton cloth and raffia palm fronds and sold them in regional markets. During the worst of the mosquito season, they also built temporary "mosquito huts" out of a tough local grass that was attached to a makeshift wooden frame. The mosquito huts were built with a small opening that could be sealed. They could be installed either outside or inside the usual living quarters and were put to use during a single mosquito season, after which they were destroyed to make room for other functions.[3]

The efficacy of these mosquito nuisance control practices was variable. The practices did not prevent the transmission of malaria, although they reduced the total infective bites received by an individual who practiced one or more forms of protection. The ongoing transmission of malaria parasites, however, meant that bouts of fever were a common occurrence in virtually all sedentary communities in tropical Africa, with the exception of those in some highland regions. Pastoral peoples, whose livelihoods required that they travel with their herds and whose living quarters were frequently makeshift, developed other practices that likewise were only partially effective against a range of insects. The Masai in East Africa, for example, smeared their bodies with sheep's fat and red ochre to repel insects.[4]

AFRICAN ANTIMALARIALS

The near universality of malarial fever across tropical Africa spurred communities everywhere to develop their own local and regional pharmacopeia. Some of this knowledge was of long-standing, as understandings of the medicinal efficacy of certain plants passed from one generation to the next. (Modern researchers have discovered that more than a thousand different plants are held to have antimalarial or anti-fever properties.) Yet Africans also borrowed freely and adopted widely. Some of the most important

---

not have a protective effect against malarial infections in 519 children who were studied in the 1980s. R. W. Snow, A. K. Bradley, R. Hayes, P. Byass, and B. M. Greenwood, "Does Woodsmoke Protect Against Malaria?," *Annals of Tropical Medicine and Parasitology*, vol. 81, no. 4 (1987), 449–451.

[3] A. Félix Iroko, *Une histoire des hommes et des moustiques en Afrique* (Paris: L'Harmattan, 1994), 76–115.

[4] J. P. de Mello, "Some Aspects of Malaria in Kenya," *East African Medical Journal*, vol. 24, no. 3 (1947), 124–125.

medicinal plants with antimalarial properties were recognized across a wide region: this was the case with the neem tree (*Azadirachta indica*). Indigenous to South and Southeast Asia, the neem tree was introduced into tropical Africa in the late nineteenth or early twentieth century, and it won a favored place in the domain of antimalarial treatments. Communities across the drylands of Africa, from Senegal to Somalia, adopted its use.[5] Other plants with protective qualities were widely embraced. A chrysanthemum species *(Chrysanthemum cinerariifolium)*, indigenous to the Balkans, was introduced to East Africa, probably also in the late nineteenth or early twentieth century, and formulations of chrysanthemum extracts containing pyrethrum became widely popular as an outdoor smudge pot fumigant and, in a more recent indoor form, as mosquito coils.

The western biomedical community had long all but ignored African antimalarials. When the standard of measure is whether or not an antimalarial medicine is capable of clearing an infection – the principal concern of Europeans in Africa – most if not all of the tropical African treatments fall short. The African therapies likely had small success in reducing childhood deaths. They were most effective for those in the post-childhood years who had already survived early mortal encounters with falciparum malaria.

For Africans who lived in environments in which one might receive hundreds of infective bites per year and in which the cause of a bout of severe fever might be ascribed variously to environmental or supernatural exposures, the goal of therapy was to find relief from the rigors of a bout of fever. Therapy was palliative, not curative. Some African antimalarials reduced an individual's parasite load in the midst of severe illness, lessened the symptoms, and thereby provided relief from suffering. Other therapies

---

[5] The leaves of the neem tree have a broad range of therapeutic actions. For recent surveys, see R. Subapriya and S. Nagini, "Medical Properties of Neem Leaves: A Review," *Current Medical Chemistry–Anti-Cancer Agents*, vol. 5, no. 2 (2005), 149–156; K. Biswas, I. Chattophadhyay, R. K. Banerjee, and U. Bandyopadhyay, "Biological Activities and Medicinal Properties of Neem (*Azadirachta indica*)," *Current Science*, vol. 82, no. 11 (2002), 1336–1345. Neem oil also has a potent antilarval action. See V. K. Dua, A. C. Pandey, K. Raghavendra, A. Gupta, T. Sharma, and A. P. Dash, "Larvicidal Activity of Neem Oil (*Azadirachta indica*) Formulation Against Mosquitoes," *Malaria Journal*, vol. 8 (2009), available online: http://www.malariajournal.com/content/8/1/124

  The history of the introduction of the neem tree to tropical Africa has been little researched. As an ad hoc committee of Board of Science and Technology for International Development noted in a 1992 publication, "earlier in this century people somehow managed to introduce this Indian tree to West Africa..." [Board on Science and Technology for International Development, National Research Council, *Neem: A Tree for Solving Global Problems* (Washington, D.C., National Academy Press, 1992), 1.]

did not have a direct action on the parasite; yet these acted as psychologically supportive placebos, and they, too, provided relief.

During the early years of the twentieth century, adult Europeans perceived that their risks from malaria were far greater than those of adult Africans. In urban areas, they could lower their risks of infection through the use of mosquito netting, quinine prophylaxis, and, in some settings, through residential segregation. In the case of infection, they depended on quinine for cure. For Europeans, this underscored the real and potential efficacy of European medicine in colonial Africa. Modernity was on the march, and, for the Europeans, one of its best expressions was the demonstrative power of modern medicine over tropical disease.

RURAL HIGHLAND MALARIA

In the highland regions in which Europeans established farms and plantations, they had important encounters with Africans that helped to shape European thinking about malaria into the mid-twentieth century. The encounters were particularly important in eastern and southern Africa, where the principal flows of Europeans were to areas deemed suitable for European farming, rather than to towns. In the "settler colonies," the political economy of colonialism favored Europeans over Africans, and where Africans had used many highland areas either for grazing their animals or for agriculture, Europeans generally got the upper hand in contests over land rights. The Europeans forced many Africans to move into newly designated "native reserves," and those who remained resident became "squatters" on lands that had formerly been their own.

In the early years of European colonialism, the highland farming areas had generally been considered to be more or less free from African fevers and thus safer for Europeans. By the 1920s, however, it became clear that the reduced vulnerability to mosquito-borne disease came at an epidemiological price. During unusually warm seasons, the ranges of the anophelines extended to higher elevations and thereby endangered both the partially immune and the nonimmune human communities; an unusually warm *and* rainy season guaranteed bountiful swarms of mosquitoes. This combustible combination occurred relatively infrequently, but it was a recipe for malaria epidemics.

When Europeans took control of these highlands, they needed to secure the services of African laborers. They found the leverage to do so in part by taking advantage of a colonial system of taxation that required African subjects to pay a head or hut tax in colonial currency that Africans could typically acquire only by working on European-owned farms. Workers were drawn from the native reserves in the highlands and from colonial lowland regions. These population movements created a stronger potential for transmission in the highlands than there had been in earlier centuries. Many of the imported laborers were parasitized, and they were settled in numbers sufficient to allow for malaria transmission.

The establishment of a European farm in the highlands thus typically created conditions conducive to the transmission of malaria. From the earliest days when a farmer first pitched his tent near a convenient water source, the frequent tramping along its banks by the farmer, the African laborers, and the farmer's oxen created habitat for anopheline breeding. The mosquitoes fed on the African laborers, many of whom were parasitized, and on the farmer; in short order, the farmer came down with debilitating fever. One solution was to impose a rural variant of residential segregation. In the highlands of Kenya, for example, farmers were recommended to have their "house boys" and other laborers sheltered at least 200 meters away from their farmhouses to reduce infiltration by infected mosquitoes.[6]

European estate owners and colonial malariologists perceived malaria to be principally a disease problem of Europeans.[7] On some plantations, they undertook environmental engineering projects to limit anopheline breeding grounds. On the coffee estates on Mount Meru, for example, estate owners had oil mixed with sawdust spread on the breeding sites of *Anopheles gambiae* and earth drains dug to empty some of the swamps. The achievements were significant, although they fell short of full control. The interventions reduced the size of the anopheline populations by more than three-quarters, and the season of transmission fell from eight or nine to two months.[8]

[6] James, *Report on a Visit to Kenya and Uganda*, 22–23, 27–29.

[7] As D. Bagster Wilson and Margaret E. Wilson put it: "As is well known to residents, the financial resources of most estates, and particularly of coffee estates, in East Africa have, during the past few years, been very limited. Any expensive schemes for the prevention of disease have therefore no possibility of general adoption. This restriction applies particularly to the case of malaria, a disease which does not cause any appreciable amount of sickness among the small African labour forces, and cannot therefore be invoked as an important cause of economic loss on their account. It is primarily and chiefly as a cause of sickness among Europeans that malaria has to be combated on estates in hyper-endemic areas." [D. Bagster Wilson and Margaret E. Wilson, "Control of *A. gambiae* on Coffee Estates," *East African Medical Journal*, vol. 16, no. 11 (1939–1940), 405.]

[8] Wilson and Wilson, "Control of *A. gambiae* on Coffee Estates," 413–415.

The generally low levels of transmission in the highlands posed risks to the Africans as well as the Europeans. The low levels of immunity in the highlands offered scant protection when workers traveled down the mountains into the lowlands. As early as 1925, the director of the medical laboratory at Kitéga in Ruanda-Urundi (now Rwanda and Burundi) discovered high death rates suffered by those who ventured some 1,400 meters down the mountain in 1925 and contracted malaria on the plains.[9] The introduction of malaria from the lowlands could have similarly devastating effects on the highland communities that stayed put. At the Belgian mission at Fataki in the Ituri region of the eastern Belgian Congo, situated at 1,500–2,000 meters, a small epidemic erupted in 1933–1934 and some sixty Africans were hospitalized. Most were adults. Even with quinine treatment, two died.[10] In 1934–1935, a larger epidemic broke out in Ruanda-Urundi in the Ngozi territory, situated at about 2,000 meters. Nearly one in seven of a population of 5,500 sought treatment and there were seventy-four deaths. A "massive usage" of quinine was launched toward the end of the epidemic, and its success led to the broader acceptance of mass chemical treatment of Africans in epidemic conditions.[11] Similar epidemics broke out in highland communities in Kenya during the 1940s.[12]

Some of the malarial epidemics were powered by the introduction of new falciparum strains to the parasite mosaic. There were, for example, different falciparum strains in Kenya, and when migrants and their families from the Elgeyo Reserve, an area of heavy endemic malaria transmission, resettled in the Turbo-Kipkarren district, they had little protection against the predominant falciparum strain there. The immigrants contracted severe infections, and cerebral malaria was common.[13]

In Southern Rhodesia (now Zimbabwe), the worst malarious regions were the fertile river valleys in which Europeans established farms. Some of

[9] G. Mattlet, "Quelques considerations sur des cas de fièvre paratyphoïde C et contribution à l'étude des bacilles paratyphoïdes," *Annales de la Société belge de medicine tropicale*, vol. 11, no. 4 (1931), 475. Kitéga is in contemporary Burundi.
[10] R. Calonne, "La malaria dans le Haut-Ituri," *Annales de la Société belge de médecine tropicale*, vol. 15, no. 4 (1935), 501–520, esp. 517.
[11] A. Duren, "Un essai d'étude d'ensemble du paludisme au Congo Belge," 19–20.
[12] de Mello, "Some Aspects of Malaria in Kenya," 112–126; J.P. de Mello, "Survey of Malaria Among the Indigenous Population in the Highlands of Kenya," *East African Medical Journal*, vol. 28, no. 11 (1951), 469.
[13] Rhodes House Library, Oxford. MSS.Afr.r.104. C.S. Pitt, "Malaria Control and Its Relation to Other Environmental Work in a European Settled Area, Kenya Colony [April 1955]," 16.

the districts were 900–1,000 meters above sea level. Experts recommended that the Europeans on these farms screen their houses and adhere strictly to mosquito net usage. The main source of infection was thought to be African children, with their high densities of gametocytes, and some experts argued for the strict residential segregation of Europeans and Africans in rural areas. Another proposal was for routine chemotherapeutic treatment of all African children at the beginning of the malarial season with euquinine (a quinine formulation without a bitter taste) or pamaquine in order to reduce the reservoir of parasites that endangered the European population.[14]

Europeans in highland towns were also considered to be at risk. P. C. C. Garnham, who had had experience with malaria control in Kisumu, Kenya, recommended the intensive treatment of the ill, treatment of parasite carriers who would be identified by blood examination, education of the African population, residential segregation, regular maintenance of drains installed to dry out the wet breeding areas, larviciding, attention to new breeding grounds that had been inadvertently created, drainage of the town proper, and the positioning of native communities between the anopheline breeding sites and the European communities. The Africans or their cattle would attract the mosquitoes and thereby protect the Europeans.[15]

Europeans were well aware that the colonization of the "White Highlands" had led to an increase in the incidence of malaria. One theory held that it was an inevitable consequence of the transport revolution.[16] Railroads and motorized vehicles wheeled the vectors hither and yon. In 1941–1944, for example, when malaria broke out at Londiani in Kenya on European farms situated between 7,500 and 8,500 feet, the vectors were thought in all likelihood to have been introduced via truck and rail.[17] The

---

[14] Comment of Dr. J. H. Moore in Thomson, "Endemic and Epidemic Malaria," 1057.
[15] Comment by Dr. J. B. Christopherson in Thomson, "Endemic and Epidemic Malaria in Southern Rhodesia," 1057.
[16] The construction of the railroad systems also complicated malaria control. In East Africa, the railroads employed large numbers of Europeans, Indians, and Africans. Many of the workers lived in close proximity to the towns and stations where they worked. The process of construction – the reconfiguration of the land to accommodate tracks and roads meant the building up of embankments and the inadvertent damming of natural drainage channels – resulted in the creation of mosquito breeding habitat. Some of these sites were intensely malarious.
[17] P. C. C. Garnham, "Malaria Epidemics at Exceptionally High Altitudes in Kenya," British Medical Journal, vol. 2, no. 4410 (14 July 1945), 45–47.

Europeans, however, saw the colonial occupation of the White Highlands as a beneficial process of modernization, and they rationalized the outbreaks of malaria as one of the unavoidable costs – an "externality" – of development rather than an indicator of underdevelopment.[18]

RURAL LOWLAND MALARIA

Europeans gained control of productive lowlands as well as highlands and thereby produced new patterns of malaria transmission. In the lowlands of Kenya, the very instance of setting up a sisal plantation, for example, created anopheline breeding habitat and thus baseline conditions for higher transmission. As the entomologist C. B. Symes noted:

Mosquito trouble on sisal estates starts from the very beginning of development. A permanent water supply is of course necessary and the factory must be placed near this. Large numbers of native labourers have to be employed and for convenience and economy their camps are built along the banks of the river. Europeans must be near their work and their staff and their residences are also placed along the river.

However free a river may be from mosquitoes it cannot possibly remain so for long under the above conditions. The factory itself often requires a dam and waste water bearing sisal wash is discharged down the hill-side; swampy conditions must arise. The water supply for hundreds of natives is the river; holes are made for washing or the better collection of drinking water, small shambas [cultivated fields and gardens] are made and attempts at irrigation started. The whole river side becomes a series of holes and ditches holding stagnant water and the river is frequently blocked by broken banks or accumulations of deposited refuse.[19]

[18] See, for example, P. C. C. Garnham, "The Incidence of Malaria at High Altitudes," *Journal of the National Malaria Society*, vol. 7, no. 4 (1948), 276. Garnham continued to champion this view into the late 1960s: "The accelerated development of these territories, which began after World War I, was accompanied by a diffusion of malaria. The railways and roads transported A. *gambiae* and A. *funestus* from the malarious lowlands into the hills, where the ubiquitous borrow-pits and badly drained swamps provided ideal breeding places for the respective mosquitoes. Malaria-infected African immigrants moved into this formerly healthy region and conditions became set for epidemics at intervals, which have recurred ever since." [P. C. C. Garnham, "The Changing Pattern of Disease in East Africa," *East African Medical Journal*, vol. 45, no. 10 (1968), 642.]

[19] Symes, "Anophelines and Malaria in Kenya," 167. Symes was struck by the fact that the estate managers had no sense of the economic costs of malaria to their enterprises and that there was no method for recording sickness among the African laboring population, which could number 1,000 on a sisal estate.

D. Bagster Wilson thought that the problem of malaria on the sisal estates was principally owing to the introduction of laborers from the Rundi or Ha ethnic groups who were

In parts of lowland West Africa in which malaria transmission was heavy, some Europeans saw that there was money to be made in setting up plantations, even though the prospects for malaria control were difficult. On the Firestone Rubber Plantation in Liberia, for example, malariologists determined that the high levels of infection among laborers and the high densities of anophelines rendered the usual malaria control methods impractical. In the early 1930s, they administered plasmochin, which destroyed gametocytes in the blood, to two camps of laborers to determine the possibility of reducing the percentage of infected anopheline mosquitoes. It was not intended to clear the parasite infections: the goal was to reduce the infectiousness of African workers to the mosquitoes with the hope that this would lower rates of transmission. The initial findings were that the intervention had lowered the rates of infected anophelines, and the malariologists recommended a second trial over a wider area and for a longer period of time to determine the feasibility of mass drug administration as a malaria intervention.[20] In their view, however, the prospects were for only limited success. The malariologists judged that Firestone would have to deal with the issue of highly infected laborers into the foreseeable future. They suggested a more balanced diet for the laborers to reduce the parasite rate.[21]

On the Firestone holdings, chemical therapies seemed promising to the malariologists of the 1930s because large-scale environmental engineering programs to reduce mosquito habitat were expensive and not always technically feasible, and larviciding was judged to be of limited utility.[22] Mosquito control was expensive. It had to compete with other financial priorities, and it could be fraught with unanticipated consequences. In Freetown, mosquito control with larvicides had been greatly successful in

---

subject to severe infections. Bagster Wilson counseled simply that "[t]he remedy is evidently to avoid such tribes for labour." [Wellcome Unit for the History of Medicine, Oxford. Malaria Room. East African Malaria. Primary. Private Papers 2. D. Bagster Wilson, "Report on a Medical Survey of Sisal Estates 1939," 7.]

[20] Marshall A. Barber, Justus B. Rice, and James Y. Brown, "Malaria Studies on the Firestone Rubber Plantation in Liberia, West Africa," *American Journal of Hygiene*, vol. 15, no. 3 (1932), 621–622.

[21] Barber, Rice, and Brown, "Malaria Studies on the Firestone Rubber Plantation," 633.

[22] Marshall Barber, the Rockefeller Foundation malariologist who led the Firestone study, had carried out antilarval experiments in Lagos and Yaba in southern Nigeria and also had considerable experience in Freetown, Sierra Leone. In his judgment, larvicides in West Africa could do little more than act as adjuvants to environmental engineering projects. More substantial results would come through drainage and filling of swamps. See M. A. Barber, "Malaria Control Work in West Africa," *Southern Medical Journal*, vol. 25, no. 6 (1932), 650.

reducing clinical disease. In the immediate post-Second World War period, the vector mosquito densities were kept low, but the parasite rate in the African population rose as a result of an increase in malaria among adults who had lost their immunities.[23]

Along the southern frontier of tropical Africa, African workers who sought employment on European farms and estates entered dangerous malarial environments. From what is today Swaziland and the Limpopo, Gauteng, North-West, KwaZulu-Natal, and Free State Provinces of South Africa, African laborers migrated to European farms and estates in search of work, particularly after the South African Land Act of 1913 stripped them of their land rights and reserved approximately 87 percent of all arable land in South Africa for Europeans.[24]

On the sugar estates, in particular, the environments could prove deadly, particularly from the late 1920s until the mid 1930s, when epidemic malaria episodically ripped through those Zulu communities that were drawn into sugar estate work. The epidemics took the form of summer outbreaks. They were remarkable because they were lethal even for adults, suggesting either that adults encountered new strains of falciparum malaria or that the previous levels of transmission were so low that there was a substantial nonimmune population. At its worst, in 1931–1932, the epidemics killed an estimated 10,000 people in Kwa-Zulu-Natal. White South Africans tried to limit the epidemic using standard methods. Antilarval interventions proved relatively ineffective. Quinine distribution was likewise unable to reduce the horrific transmission. In extremis, the authorities innovated: they sprayed the insides of houses with pyrethrum insecticide (extracted from chrysanthemums) and had remarkable success. G. A. Park Ross, the South African malariologist who pioneered the indoor vector control strategy and reported on the efforts to control the epidemics, noted that it was with unease that the insecticides were sprayed so extensively. The fear was that the intervention might impair the acquired immunity of the African populations and thus leave them more vulnerable in the future.[25]

---

[23] WHO/MAL/196. AFRO/MAL/1. 7 February 1958. "Rapport de la Réunion Technique sur le Paludisme en Afrique Occidentale," 14.

[24] On Swaziland, see Randall M. Packard, "Maize, Cattle, and Mosquitoes: The Political Economy of Malaria Epidemics in Colonial Swaziland," *Journal of African History*, vol. 25, no. 2 (1984), 189–212.

[25] G. A. Park Ross, "Insecticide as a Major Measure in the Control of Malaria, Being an Account of the Methods and Organisation Put in Force in Natal and Zululand during the Past Six Years," *Quarterly Bulletin of the Health Organisation of the League of Nations*, vol. 5 (1936), 116.

IN SOUTH AFRICA: A FIRST STEP IN INDOOR
VECTOR CONTROL

The indoor vector control strategy in South Africa was based on spraying the walls and ceilings of human habitations with pyrethrum insecticides to kill adult mosquitoes. Pyrethrum insecticides worked well, but their killing powers dissipated quickly. Walls and ceilings had to be resprayed frequently to reduce the transmission of malaria, and this proved too expensive for use in other than epidemic emergencies. Yet the early experiences with indoor spraying seemed technically promising, and, in 1935, at the Pan-African Health Conference in Johannesburg, experts called for further experiments.

The malaria problem was somewhat different in South Africa than in tropical Africa, but malarial control efforts there shared some common features with those in the African tropics. These efforts focused on the drainage and filling-in of mosquito habitat and the use of larvicides on surface waters. The European community reserved the use of quinine as a prophylactic and curative drug principally to themselves. The major exception, authorized by the Transvaal government in the late 1930s, was for the free distribution of quinine to Africans in the event of an epidemic.[26] The goal of the control efforts was to protect the health of Europeans and of those Africans who worked on European farms and plantations and in the mines or who lived in cities and large towns with sizeable European populations. Europeans saw that malarial infections undermined African worker morale and productivity, and where African workers or urban dwellers lived in close proximity to Europeans, the health of the Africans was perceived as directly relevant to the health of Europeans. Otherwise, it was not. In rural Africa, during the depths of the global economic depression, the Pan-African Health Conference committee saw that the only realistic prospects for large-scale antimalaria interventions were those that could be linked to increases in Africans' standards of living. Investments to improve African nutrition and housing should accompany any antimalaria efforts, and, indeed, the success of the antimalaria efforts might well depend upon them.[27]

---

[26] I am grateful to Randy Packard for this information.

[27] [Pan-African Health Conference], "Malaria under African Conditions," *Quarterly Bulletin of the Health Organisation of the League of Nations*, vol. 5 (1936), 110–113; Annex I, G. A. Park Ross, "Insecticide as a Major Measure in the Control of Malaria," 114–133; and Annex II, B. De Meillon, "The Control of Malaria in South Africa by Measures Directed against the Adult Mosquitoes in Habitations," *Quarterly Bulletin of the Health Organisation of the League of Nations*, vol. 5 (1936), 134–137.

The early pyrethrum spraying experiences were a major influence on later control efforts within tropical Africa, yet specialists soon recognized that there were important ecological differences between the subtropical southern African region and the core regions of tropical Africa. The southern African vectors were dangerous – particularly *Anopheles funestus* and *An. arabiensis* – but the region did not have to contend with a heavy presence of *An. gambiae sensu stricto*, a principal vector elsewhere in sub-Saharan Africa; and in the subtropics, malaria transmission was decidedly seasonal rather than year-round.[28]

NEW THERAPEUTIC APPROACHES

What was the appropriate role for antimalarial drugs in treating Africans? Across the colonies, there were experiments to treat Africans with quinine and occasionally with plasmochin, a drug that killed falciparum gametocytes, as well as alleviated suffering.[29] There were two principal constraints. One was financial – the antimalarial drugs were expensive. The other was the belief that treating Africans might do them more harm than good because the drugs might compromise their acquired immunity.

In the Gold Coast, the British undertook some early experiments with preventive quinine therapy for school-age children. In 1910, the British authorities in Accra distributed quinine coated with chocolate to schoolchildren, but the chocolate didn't mask the intense bitterness of the quinine and most of the children threw it away. Further efforts to provide quinine to schoolchildren in the Gold Coast were made sporadically in 1919 and the early 1920s, but again without much success. In 1935, authorities began to make quinine for curative purposes available to the general population who lived near one of the 270 Post Offices in the colony. The authorities sold at cost 36,000 tubes of sixteen quinine tablets of four grains, each tablet grooved so that it could be split into doses appropriate for children. Sales doubled in two years. In 1937, the program was extended to the Northern Territories of the Gold Coast through the Native Authorities. The program continued into the Second World War,

---

[28] For the distribution of malarial vectors in tropical Africa, see Jean Mouchet et al., *Biodiversité du paludisme dans le monde*, 66–75; for the entomology of Mozambique, Zimbabwe, Swaziland, Namibia, and South Africa, see 158–167.

[29] Physicians' awareness of the toxic side effects of plasmochin grew only gradually during the 1930s. See Leo B. Slater, *War and Disease: Biomedical Research on Malaria in the Twentieth Century* (New Brunswick: Rutgers University Press, 2009), 66–68.

when prices for quinine rose and the distribution of antimalarials was shifted to medical dispensaries.[30] A similar program of distribution developed in Nigeria. Quinine was also offered at a cost price through the Post Offices in tubes containing sixteen four-grain tablets, and quinine purchases grew from 1,461 pounds in 1934 to 2,250 pounds in 1937.[31]

Elsewhere in the British colonies, experiences diverged. The Uganda Protectorate estimated that the free issue of quinine from hospitals and dispensaries reached 20 percent of the total population.[32] By contrast, in Sierra Leone, most of the population had little or no contact with European medicine,[33] and in Nyasaland (now Malawi), only "a very small proportion" of malaria cases received quinine treatment.[34] In Tanganyika (now mainland Tanzania), the total sales of quinine went to treat some 41,000 non-Africans.[35]

In French tropical Africa, the provision of quinine was principally reserved to Europeans. There were experiments with the "quininization" of some African schoolchildren in Madagascar, Sénégal, Gabon, and Réunion and a few hundred children in the development zone in Mali called the Office du Niger.[36] These remained small-scale affairs, continuing into the immediate post-Second World War period. The Portuguese likewise restricted the use of quinine to those who were under the care of physicians, and this was a predominantly European and Luso-African clientele.

In Belgian Africa, the provision of quinine was also fairly limited. In the Belgian Congo, during the 1920s and early 1930s, among the community of 1,500 of so Europeans who were under the care of Western physicians, the toll from malaria had been sharply cut. Quinine, mosquito nets and screens, and environmental engineering projects had been used to good advantage. Among African colonial subjects of the Belgian Congo,

---

[30] K. David Patterson, *Health in Colonial Ghana: Disease, Medicine, and Socio-Economic Change, 1900–1955* (Waltham, MA: Crossroads Press, 1981), 35–36; NAUK, CO323/1620/5, Gold Coast. No. 476. Governor to the Secretary of State for the Colonies [n.d. (1938)].

[31] NAUK, CO323/1620/5, Nigeria. No. 679. Governor's Deputy to the Secretary of State for the Colonies, 21 July 1938.

[32] NAUK, CO323/1620/5, Uganda Protectorate. No. 218. Governor to the Secretary of State for the Colonies, 8 August 1938.

[33] NAUK, CO323/1620/5, Sierra Leone, No. 440. 13 July 1938.

[34] NAUK, CO323/1620/5, Nyasaland. No. 285. 30 June 1938.

[35] NAUK, CO323/1620/5, Tanganyika Territory, No. 346, Governor to the Secretary of State, 24 June 1938.

[36] M. Vaucel, "Etat actuel du paludisme dans les colonies françaises," *Bullétin de la Société de pathologie exotique et de ses filiales*, vol. 39, nos. 1–2 (1946), 33.

however, the malarial toll was coming into view. A. Duren, director of the Belgian colonial health service and former medical hygiene inspector in the Belgian Congo, collated and analyzed a number of medical surveys of indigenous malaria and concluded that malaria was a major cause of death and disease for Africans.[37] The overall childhood death rates were high, and many deaths were attributed to malaria, although determining the actual cause of death was an inexact science. Virtually all children who died were parasitized, and all children who survived were parasitized.

One therapeutic approach was discovered through trial and error and determined to be highly effective, although the reasons for its success were uncertain. European physicians in the Belgian Congo discovered that irregular quinine doses administered to African children cut their mortality rate by 50 percent. This was such a spectacular intervention that it became a normal practice in the Belgian Congo, although the number of Africans who came within the orbit of European physicians was small.[38] As Duren put it in his mid-1930s review article on malaria in the Belgian colonies: "All of the [malaria specialist] authors [in the Belgian colonies] are unanimous in their view that the regular administration of quinine, particularly to native children, considerably diminishes the proportion of acute bouts of malaria and makes the bouts that do occur more benign. The impact of this treatment on disease symptoms is uncontested. All of the authors also hold that children treated with quinine have better general health."[39]

Interestingly, the Belgian experience in the Congo also brought to light the fact that chemotherapeutic treatment was differentially effective against malaria parasites. Treatment of small cohorts of African children at Stanleyville in the Belgian Congo demonstrated that quinine suppressed malariae infections much more effectively than falciparum infections. It

---

[37] Duren, "Un essai d'étude d'ensemble du paludisme au Congo Belge," 7–18.

[38] Duren, "Un essai d'étude d'ensemble du paludisme au Congo Belge," 65–66.

[39] "Disons immédiatement que tous les auteurs sont unanimes à déclarer que l'adminstration régulière de quinine, notamment à des enfants indigenes, diminue dans des proportions très considerables le nombre des accès du paludisme febrile et rend également plus bénins les accès qui surviennent. L'influence sur les manifestations du paludisme "maladie apparente" est donc incontestée. Tous les auteurs constatent également chez les enfants quininisés une meilleure santé générale." [Duren, "Un essai d'étude d'ensemble du paludisme au Congo Belge," 65.]

Blood transfusions were used in the Belgian Congo to treat infants with anemia caused by malaria. The first blood transfusion for this purpose was reported in 1939, and, from 1943 through 1951, a systematic treatment program completed more than 5,700 transfusions at an average of four per patient. Transfusion for malaria treatment was replaced by nivaquine treatment in the 1950s. [William H. Schneider, *A History of Blood Transfusion in Sub-Saharan Africa* (Athens: Ohio University Press, 2013).]

confirmed some of the malariological evidence from North Africa that showed that chemical treatment might transform the parasite mosaics, producing a greater predominance of falciparum infections.[40]

Although the effectiveness of treating parasitized African children with quinine had been demonstrated, government authorities in the tropical African colonies were wary of a general public health initiative. Most medical experts thought that treatment had to be advanced in a way that took account of acquired immunity, but just how to do so remained uncertain. Perhaps it was best to treat only truly severe cases. As the director of medical services on Zanzibar put it: "It is important not to disturb the full and rapid development of this tolerance until it is possible to prevent infection, a state of affairs which is not within sight yet. At the same time, the treatment of acute attacks particularly in the early years of life, would save a great many lives."[41] Some medical authorities counseled that a public health initiative might be dangerous for the adult African population. As the acting governor of Northern Rhodesia put it: "I am advised that the indiscriminate use of quinine by Africans is open to objection as it is apt to destroy their natural immunity to malaria."[42]

Quite apart from the issue of the potential destruction of acquired immunity was that of the sheer quantity of antimalarial alkaloids that would be required. In Tanganyika, medical experts estimated that the "younger half" of the more than 5 million Africans in the territory would benefit from curative treatment, preferably with cinchonine and cinchonidine (cinchona alkaloids that were far less expensive than quinine), and cautioned that the requirements of the "partially immune" were

---

[40] J. Schwetz, "Le 'mystère' de la fièvre quarte et de la tierce bénigne en Afrique Equatoriale et Centrale," *Bulletin de la Société de Pathologie exotique*, vol. 25 (1932), 1071. Schwetz's finding confirmed that of French researchers in Morocco. [C. Vialatte and P. E. Flye Sainte-Marie, "Autour du 'Mystère' de la fièvre quarte," *Bulletin de la Société de Pathologie exotique et de ses filiales*, vol. 24 (1931), 282.]

Some researchers have advanced evidence for a density-dependent regulation of mixed malaria parasite infections in humans and suggested that interventions that reduce the prevalence of one parasitemia could provide an increased opportunity for other species to multiply. This could result in an increase in prevalence, transmission potential, and disease. See Marian C. Bruce, Christl A. Donnelly, Michael P. Alpers, Mary R. Galinski, John W. Barnwell, David Walliker, and Karen P. Day, "Cross-Species Interactions between Malaria Parasites in Humans," *Science*, vol. 287, 4 February 2000, 845–848.

[41] NAUK, CO323/1620/5, Memorandum by the Director of Medical Services on the Consumption of Quinine in the Zanzibar Protectorate. Enclosure in the British Resident's Despatch No. 126 of 4 May 1938.

[42] NAUK, CO323/1620/5, Northern Rhodesia, No. 190, Acting Governor to the Secretary of State for the Colonies, 18 June 1938.

difficult to estimate.[43] On Zanzibar, authorities projected that the treatment of all malaria attacks would require a twenty-fold increase in quinine dispensations.[44]

CINCHONA PLANTATIONS IN TROPICAL AFRICA

The sheer expense of quinine militated against its use at the population level.[45] One promising approach was to grow cinchona trees in the colonies and prepare a therapeutic mixture of the alkaloids, without undertaking the more costly procedure of isolating quinine.[46] This was easier said than done, however, because the cinchona trees could be grown only in specialized ecological zones, at elevations of 1,500 meters or more. The European imperial powers embarked in their African colonies on modest efforts to grow cinchona and achieved modest results.

The Portuguese planted cinchona in Angola and on the island of São Tomé with minor success. The British did the same in Tanganyika.[47] The Belgians, after some false starts, deemed a site in the Ituri highland region in the northeast of the Belgian Congo to be suitable for cinchona, and workers put thousands of seedlings in the ground in the mid-1930s.[48] The French provided some intermittent financial support to government

[43] NAUK, CO323/1620/5, Tanganyika Territory, No. 346, Governor to the Secretary of State, 24 June 1938.

[44] NAUK, CO323/1620/5, Memorandum by the Director of Medical Services on the Consumption of Quinine in the Zanzibar Protectorate. Enclosure in the British Resident's Despatch No. 126 of 4 May 1938.

[45] Global quinine production was concentrated on the island of Java in the Dutch East Indies. There, European-run plantations were vertically integrated. They grew cinchona trees, processed the bark, sold the quinine, recovered their expenses, and made normal profits. A Dutch government-authorized Kina Bureau headquartered in Amsterdam set prices. Cinchona was hard to grow and quinine was expensive to isolate. The drug remained beyond the means of the impoverished who suffered from malaria, and it was far less expensive than the best available alternative. Atebrine, a synthetic antimalarial drug developed by the Germans and produced under a monopoly of manufacture, cost nearly five times as much per course of therapeutic treatment as did quinine.

[46] This approach had been followed in India since the late nineteenth century. Webb, *Humanity's Burden*, 151.

[47] Jean-Louis Gramont, "Le paludisme," *Marchés coloniaux*, novembre 1947, 1683; Jean-Paul Bado, "La lutte contre le paludisme en Afrique central. Problèmes d'hier et d'aujourd'hui," *Enjeux*, no. 18, janvier-mars 2004, 11.

[48] Duren, "Un essai d'étude d'ensemble du paludisme au Congo Belge," 61. There was considerable irony in this. The highland region of Ituri was at an elevation that, before the arrival of Belgian coffee planters earlier in the century, had inhibited the transmission of malaria. When the coffee planters moved into the highlands, they built small dams to provision themselves with enough water to process their coffee beans and, in the process,

cinchona plantations in Cameroon and Madagascar. Yet what could be achieved was extremely modest. Cinchona production in tropical Africa paled into near insignificance when compared with the better successes in British India and French Indochina, for which the groundwork had been laid in earlier decades.[49] The global economic depression of the 1930s and the outbreak of the Second World War restricted investments of all kinds in the colonies, and, in this respect, the cinchona initiative fell victim to poor timing.

THE ISSUE OF ADULT AFRICAN IMMUNITY

Over the first three decades of the twentieth century, malariologists sought new understanding of the immunities of adult Africans that seemed to protect them from frequent manifestations of disease. This search was undergirded by the discoveries of the high rates of parasitization among African children and the far lower rates among African adults, as revealed by spleen rates, and high parasite densities in African children and far lower parasite densities in African adults, as revealed through the microscopic study of blood smears.

Were African immunities the same as European immunities? With regard to European immunity, physicians were agreed that it was won after surviving a number of bouts of the disease. This was in accord with long-standing observations about the "seasoning" of adult nonimmunes

---

created shallow pools of water that extended over several hectares. These became the breeding habitat for vector mosquitoes. The Ituri coffee highlands became highly malarious in the lands immediately surrounding the dams. Even the draining of the swampy low points in the highlands to create new coffee fields proved to be an epidemiological disaster. These wetlands kept night temperatures 4 to 6 degrees Centigrade lower than did the drained lands. The colder temperatures were hard on the coffee bushes, but after drainage, the low points became warm enough to serve as anopheline breeding habitat during the hot season. See R. Calonne, "La malaria dans le Haut-Ituri," 501–520.

[49] Within British India, cinchona alkaloids were produced on government plantations and the volume was never sufficient to meet demand; British India imported cinchona alkaloids from Java. [J. M. Cowan, "Cinchona in the Empire," *Empire Forestry Journal*, vol. 8, no. 1 (1929), 45–53.] By 1940, French Indochina was self-sufficient in quinine and exported some to Madagascar. [IMTSSA, Box 232 (n.a.), "La lutte contre le paludisme dans nos colonies," 2, 9–10. (1944); IMTSSA, Box 232. Dossiers Antipaludiques. M. Robert, M. le Médecin Général Inspecteur, Directeur Général de la Santé Publique en A.O.F. à M. le Directeur des Affaires Economiques et du Plan [received 14 November 1955], 1.]

For a global overview, see M. Kerbosch, "Some Notes on Cinchona Culture and the World Consumption of Quinine," *Bulletin of the Colonial Institute of Amsterdam*, vol. 3, no. 1 (1939), 36–51.

who were introduced into malarial environments in the Mediterranean region, the Americas, or Asia.

In tropical Africa, however, the European experiences seemed different. As early as 1901, C. W. Daniels observed that Europeans in Central Africa who survived their initial encounters did acquire a partial immunity to malaria, yet this partial immunity seemed to be accompanied by further grave dangers. The longer that Europeans stayed in tropical Africa, the more prone they seemed to be to "blackwater fever." This view became a part of general European medical knowledge about malaria before the Second World War. J. G. Thomson underscored this point in his 1933 review of studies on malarial immunity: "Acquired immunity in Europeans, at least, is far from satisfactory and may be highly dangerous." By contrast, blackwater fever seemed to be practically unknown in African children. This suggested that the process of immunity might have a racial component.[50]

There was no general agreement on the issue, but some support for this proposition could be evinced from studies conducted in the 1930s – well before the mid-twentieth-century revolution in molecular science – that indicated that people of African descent were less susceptible than people of European descent to vivax malaria. The racial interpretation – in the era before the discovery of Duffy antigen negativity – raised important questions. If Africans had a different kind of immunity than did Europeans, should they receive the same kind of medical treatment? Or might medical treatment do more harm than good by degrading or reversing the immunological status of the Africans?[51]

Malariologists judged malaria in African adults to be relatively mild; and, for many experts, this suggested the need for prudence. Some argued that there was no need to undertake any population-level intervention. This view meshed well with the constraints posed by the high cost and limited supply of quinine. It was further reinforced by the view of some prominent malariologists that the chemotherapeutic treatment of African

[50] J. G. Thomson, "Immunity in Malaria," *Transactions of the Royal Society of Tropical Medicine and Hygiene*, vol. 26, no. 6 (1933), 484, 499.

[51] The issue of the acquired immunity of tropical Africans had purchase beyond sub-Saharan Africa. French colonial troops in Morocco were given a daily course of quinine treatment for the six months of the malaria transmission season. The exceptions were the "Sénégalais," a broad descriptor that agglomerated Black African troops of different ethnic groups from across the French West African colonies who were held to be barely susceptible to malarial infection. [Vialatte and Flye Sainte-Marie, "Autour du 'Mystère,'" 282.]

adults might constitute a profound disservice to them, in that the therapy might weaken their immune status and make them more vulnerable to bouts of severe malaria and blackwater fever.

The question of whether to treat adult Africans for malaria thus was directly bound up with the conundrum of acquired immunity. Malariologists knew that there was considerable variation in the severity of disease symptoms among individuals who suffered malarial infections, and this might well mean that there was considerable variation in immune responses. Perhaps more empirical research would point the way forward. The Pan-African Health Conference of 1935 called for study of the "influence of occasional drug treatment on immunity and particularly the question whether there is any danger to a primitive community in such treatment."[52]

If adult Africans had acquired immunity to malaria, did malaria nonetheless constitute a significant health problem? In East Africa, there was a remarkable lack of accord on this question, even into the post-Second World War years. As a team of visiting expert malariologists reported on the situation in Kenya in 1950:

Malaria is taken for granted, and, except in the towns, does not appear to arouse the interest of the public health authorities who, therefore, are very poorly informed. There was for example, a remarkable divergence of opinion between two senior health officers as to the importance of malaria in a particular rural area, very well known to both; one replied that for him malaria in that area was not more important than the common cold; the other said that malaria, in that very area, represented the most debilitating disease and occupied the greatest percentage of beds in the hospitals.[53]

Many malariologists were of the opinion that African adults were not at risk for severe disease – as long as they remained in those zones of endemic infection in which they had acquired their malarial immunities. This paradigm of Africans rooted in their natal communities conflicted with colonial economic programs working to increase export-oriented production. The programs encouraged the movement of African laborers into economically productive zones, and the migrations frequently brought workers into contact with new malarial environments. In the case of laborers from nonendemic highlands, it meant the movement of the

[52] Pan-African Health Conference, "Malaria under African Conditions," 113.
[53] NAUK, CO 822/512, "Extract from a Report on a Study Tour in Central and East Africa, Dec. 1950–Jan. 1951 by Major General Sir Gordon Covell, Dr. Paul F. Russell, and Dr. E. J. Pampana."

nonimmune or partially immune into areas of intense transmission. Even Africans who were in zones of hyperendemic infection might find themselves in environments in which there were malaria genotypes to which they had little protection. Many malariologists thought that the estate and plantation owners who employed migrant laborers thus had a responsibility to select their workers on the basis of their acquired immunity or to undertake significant – and often expensive – measures to reduce transmission on their estates. There, the goal would be to reduce the incidence of severe illness, not "cure" the patient. To do so might be dangerous.

Other malariologists looked to the experience of Africans who left zones of endemic infection and returned after their immunities had degraded. Malcolm Watson noted the experience of those Black African soldiers in the Egyptian army who hailed from hyperendemic areas and served in dry, northern Sudan where there was no malaria. When they returned to the south, they succumbed to malaria. They had lost their acquired immunity, suffered epidemic malaria, and reacquired their immunity after six months.[54] What were the costs of the reacquisition of a more robust immunological status? No one knew. Could the experiences of Black African soldiers in the Egyptian army be reasonably taken to represent the experiences of tropical Africans? No one knew. Professional opinion rested upon supposition and anecdote.

THE QUESTION OF CHILDHOOD VULNERABILITY

The other major issue that bedeviled health discussions about malaria was the extent and severity of the disease in African children. An influential study in the early 1930s compared malarial infections among the native populations in the Dutch East Indies and South Africa. They concluded that infant mortality was high in the Dutch East Indies and very low among Black Africans ("Bantus"). The authors deemed that the differences were so stark that they postulated two different "types" of immunities that seemed to be based on race.[55] (These views were subjective. Later empirical

---

[54] Comment of Malcolm Watson in D. Bagster Wilson, "Implications of Malarial Endemicity in East Africa," *Transactions of the Royal Society of Tropical Medicine and Hygiene*, vol. 32, no. 4 (1939), 463.

[55] J. Schwetz, "Quelques considerations et réflexions sur l'immunité malarienne," *Rivista di malariologia*, vol. 13, no. 5 (1934), 670, citing W. A. P. Schüffner, N. H. Swellengrebel, S. Anneke, and B. de Meillon, "Vergleichende Untersuchungen über Malariaimmunität in Niederlandisch-Indien und Südafrika," *Zentralblatt für Bakteriologie*, 125 Band, Heft 1/2, July 1932.

studies in South Africa found high levels of childhood mortality there.) The implication was that the mortality costs of the acquisition of immunity for tropical Africans were acceptable.

Yet how high were these mortality costs? Experts agreed that malarial infections killed some African children, but no one knew how many. Some influential malariologists thought that the costs were high; others strongly disagreed. As late as 1950, some eminent malariologists, including D. Bagster Wilson, estimated that in areas of hyperendemic transmission, infant mortality was on the order of 1–2 percent in the absence of treatment and held that Africans were out of danger after 18 months of age.[56] By contrast, the French estimated that the mortality costs were quite high. They attributed to malaria 20 to 30 percent of infant deaths in Dakar, 32 percent in the development zone known as the Office du Niger, and a much higher percentage in Cameroun among infants brought to the health training centers. And they judged that these figures might underestimate the true mortality costs.[57]

At what ages were African children at risk of death in the zones of endemic transmission? Bagster Wilson held that all African infants acquired acute infections during the first six months of life and that this stage of infection was dangerous for a "comparatively short period" and was "definitely on the wane within a year." The later stages of infection posed "no danger to life."[58] This reinforced the view that population-level malaria control interventions were unnecessary. Indeed, if malaria control prevented infants from acquiring the immunity that was so valuable to them later in life, it might have an overall negative impact on their health. For Bagster Wilson and others who shared his views, in the case of a severe malarial infection in the early months of life, the point of a therapeutic intervention was to reduce the parasite load, rather than attempt a cure, in order not to jeopardize the acquisition of immunity.[59]

[56] D. Bagster Wilson, P. C. C. Garnham, and N. H. Swellengrebel, "A Review of Hyperendemic Malaria," *Tropical Diseases Bulletin*, vol. 47, no. 8 (1950), 695.
[57] Vaucel, "Etat actuel du paludisme dans les colonies françaises," 32.
[58] D. Bagster Wilson and Margaret E. Wilson, "The Manifestations and Measurement of Immunity to Malaria in Different Races," *Transactions of the Royal Society of Tropical Medicine and Hygiene*, vol. 30, no. 4 (1937), 435. The Wilsons did not subscribe to the view that the differential rates of immunity to malaria among communities were owing to innate racial tolerances. [Wilson and Wilson, "Manifestations and Measurement," 444.]
[59] D. Bagster Wilson, "Implications of Malarial Endemicity in East Africa," 437; Wellcome Unit for the History of Medicine, Oxford, Malaria Room. East African Malaria [EAM], Primary, UNICEF 8. K. W. C. Sinclair-Loutit, "East African High Commission Malaria Scheme," Paris, 5 November 1953, 3–5.

This was in line with the empirical experience of physicians in the Belgian colonies who had pioneered revolutionary understandings of the beneficial effects of intermittent therapeutic quinine treatment of children. The therapy could be administered even when the child was not ill because the goal of intermittent treatment was not a radical clearing of parasites or even the suppression of malaria symptoms. As Duren noted: "Regular and ongoing preventive treatment is effective; it acts without question to reduce overall morbidity and mortality and has a beneficial influence on endemic infections; it does seem not to prevent the acquisition of acquired immunity."[60]

WHAT COULD BE DONE FOR THE AFRICANS?

The global economic depression of the 1930s and the privations of the wartime years meant that malaria treatment and control efforts were scant for the African subjects of the European empires.[61] In the immediate postwar period, with quinine in short supply, Dr. Vaucel, the chief French colonial medical officer, urged that special attention be directed to ensure that quinine was used to treat infants who were at serious medical risk from malarial infections.[62] In his view, there was little hope for effective mosquito control in rural Africa. The best that could be hoped for were improvements in the malaria status of the urban centers, European neighborhoods, and African urban settlements. Those improvements would depend on the creation of a competent public health service in the colonies.[63] The financial strictures of the immediate post-Second

[60] "La medication preventive régulière et continue est un moyen efficace; elle agit incontestablement sur la morbidité et la mortalité générale, elle a une influence heureuse sur l'endémie malarienne; il semble bien qu'elle n'empêche pas la premonition de s'installer." Duren, "Un essai d'étude d'ensemble du paludisme au Congo Belge," 72.

[61] Mosquito nets, long deployed to advantage by Europeans in Africa, were coming into increasing use in parts of rural Africa by the mid 1940s, but for the most part the nets were reserved for men, who reportedly put them to use during afternoon naps, when anophelines were not active. The nets undoubtedly helped the men to rest with less annoyance from various insects, but the nets had little impact on the transmission of malaria. Indeed, the insides of the nets were said to the best place to locate anophelines that had taken their blood meals. [Vaucel, "État actuel du paludisme," 34.]

[62] Vaucel, "État actuel du paludisme," 34.

[63] Vaucel, "État actuel du paludisme," 35. The French had long taken the lead in the attempts to determine the extent of African endemic diseases and, when possible, to extend the benefits of preventive medicine. The Services d'Hygiène Mobile, an outgrowth of the Service de Santé des Troupes Coloniales, in the years following World War I carried out surveys of rural populations in order to come to a determination of the major diseases and then attempted to prioritize interventions on the basis of known, and economically feasible, methods. Dr. Eugène Jamot, on the basis of surveys carried out in the early and

World War period were severe, however, and requests from the colonial public health authorities to set up an antimalarial service fell on deaf ears in Paris. The French came to the grim conclusion that there was little to be done.[64]

Yet a new era of synthetic antimalarial drugs and synthetic insecticides was dawning. These new tools offered the promise of effective and inexpensive malaria control without causing blackwater fever.[65] The Americans and then the British were to take the lead, and the logic of the new malaria control tools soon morphed into a campaign for the eradication of the disease.

mid-1930s came to the view that sleeping sickness (trypanosomiasis) was the principal health problem for which an intervention was possible, and this was the health focus until 1939, when the French created an autonomous organization devoted exclusively to trypanosomiasis. Le Service Général d'Hygiène Mobile et de Prophylaxie was formed in 1945 and a special malaria unit at Bobo Dioulasso in Upper Volta (Burkina Faso). On the organizational history, see L. Sanner and A. Masseguin, "Le Service d'Hygiène Mobile et son oeuvre," *Bulletin médical de l'Afrique Occidentale Française*, special issue, January 1954, 9–59.

[64] As the General Instructions for the A. E. F. put it:

La conjuncture financière actuelle ne nous permet pas encore de concevoir une organisation suffisament cohérente et suffisament équipée pour fair face à toutes les incidences que réclamerait une action très largement appliquée à toutes les situations locales ou régionales des quatres territoires de l'A. E. F.

Le financement d'une telle lutte, même réduite, dépassant de beaucoup le cadre de possibilités budgétaires de la Fédération, de comité Directeur du Plan FIDES à Paris a bien voulu envisager favorablement, non seulement des investissements pour la mise en place et pour le premier équipement d'un service antipaludique mais encore, des crédits pour l'achat d'une certaine quantité de produits insecticides et de chimio-prophylactiques. Mais il s'est absolument refusé à financer le fonctionnement complet de ce service malgré tous les arguments fournis lors de la présentation d'un premier programme plus complet qui lui avait été soumis.

C'est là une des raisons qui nous ont amené à réduire nos ambitions devant les charges que ce fonctionnement impliquait et qui ont conditionné une programme d'action plus modeste pour lequel nous nous trouvons dans l'obligation de demander aux Territoires une part de collaboration.

[IMTSSA, Box 234. Gouvernement Générale de l'A. O. F. Direction Générale de la Santé Publique. Instruction Générale sur l'Organisation d'une Lutte Contre le Paludisme et sur l'Application qui Peut en Etre Faite Actuellement en Afrique Equatoriale Française, Brazzaville, 10 November 1950, 2.]

[65] The French had learned through experiments with mass chemical prophylaxis that quinine could cause blackwater fever in Africans, and they believed that quinine prophylaxis caused a dangerous loss of acquired immunity. [IMTSSA, Box 232. Le Médecin Général Inspecteur, Directeur Général de la Santé Publique en A. O. F., "Note au sujet de: La quinine dans la lutte anti-palustre en A. O. F.," 1–3.]

3

An Aborted Campaign for Eradication

In the aftermath of the Second World War, technical prospects for the control of malaria appeared promising. The success of antimalaria interventions in the southern states of the United States, Mexico, and war-ravaged Italy – in zones of mixed vivax, malariae, and falciparum infections – encouraged malariologists to expand their use of synthetic insecticides to other malarious areas.[1] Dichloro-diphenyl-trichloroethane (DDT), in particular, promised an inexpensive method of vector control and raised the prospect of effective public health interventions without having to create public health systems. At the time, this seemed to be the essence of public health economy. Enthusiasms ran high. In the immediate postwar period, malaria control campaigns were launched in Greece, Corsica, Venezuela, and Ceylon (now Sri Lanka). In 1946, the Rockefeller Foundation launched a research program on the island of Sardinia to eradicate *Anopheles labranchiae*, the principal indigenous vector there, using DDT. Over the next several years, the Rockefeller program, unable to achieve vector eradication, changed its approach and took up the banner of the first-ever campaign of disease eradication.[2]

---

[1] On the Italian experience, see Frank M. Snowden, *The Conquest of Malaria: Italy, 1900–1962* (New Haven, CT: Yale University Press, 2006), 181–197; on the U. S. experience, Margaret Humphreys, "Kicking a Dying Dog: DDT and the Demise of Malaria in the American South," *Isis*, vol. 87, no. 1 (1996), 1–17; on the Mexican experience, Darwin H. Stapleton, "The Dawn of DDT and Its Experimental Use by the Rockefeller Foundation in Mexico, 1943–1952," *Parassitologia*, vol. 40 (1998), 149–158.

[2] Eugenia Tognotti, "Program to Eradicate Malaria in Sardinia, 1946–1950," *Emerging Infectious Diseases*, vol. 15, no. 9 (2009), 1460–1466; Peter J. Brown, "Failure as Success: Multiple Meanings of Eradication in the Rockefeller Foundation Sardinia Project," *Parassitologia*, vol. 40 (1998), 117–130.

Some malariologists were cautious about the prospects in tropical Africa. They understood that the African malaria problem was different and likely more tenacious. The principal African mosquito vectors were highly efficient; in the warm, humid African tropics, they fed and reproduced year-round; and they took most of their blood meals from human beings, rather than from domesticated livestock or animals in the wild.

Yet there were grounds for optimism. Malariologists had rung up two major successes in species eradication against an African vector, albeit outside of its endemic environments. In late 1929 or early 1930, a female *An. arabiensis* traveled aboard a fast French destroyer carrying mail across the Atlantic from Dakar to northeastern Brazil and triggered a local malaria epidemic in Natal that peaked in 1931.[3] In the period 1932–1937, the African vector continued to spread in northeastern Brazil, and, in 1938–1939, a large-scale epidemic erupted. Fred L. Soper and D. Bruce Wilson of the Rockefeller Foundation countered the anopheline invasion. They imposed a military-style discipline on the Brazilian antimalaria teams and achieved "species eradication" through extensive larviciding and house-spraying, thus eliminating the African vector from Brazil. The plasmodia, however, continued to be transmitted by the less-efficient indigenous anopheline mosquitoes.[4]

During the Second World War, malariologists scored a second important victory. In the early 1940s, *An. gambiae s.s.*, introduced from south of the Sahara, ignited a malarial conflagration in Egypt that resulted in the deaths of between 100,000 and 200,000 people. As in Brazil, an aggressive larviciding program – in which Soper again played a significant role – successfully disrupted the breeding of the anopheline invader. By 1945, the Egyptian outbreak had been fully suppressed, and *An. gambiae s.s.*

[3] Fred L. Soper and D. Bruce Wilson, *Anopheles gambiae in Brazil, 1930 to 1940* (New York: The Rockefeller Foundation, 1943), 22–23.
[4] Soper and Wilson, *Anopheles gambiae*. On the deeper historical contextualization of the RF achievement in Brazil, see R. M. Packard and P. Gadelha, "A Land Filled with Mosquitoes: Fred L. Soper, the Rockefeller Foundation, and the *Anopheles gambiae* Invasion of Brazil," *Parassitologia*, vol. 36 (1994), 197–213.

In 2008, molecular investigations revealed that the African vector introduced to Brazil was *Anopheles arabiensis* not *An. gambiae*, as had long been held. [Aristides Parmakelis, Michael A. Russello, Adalgisa Caccone, Carlos Brsiola Marcondes, Jane Costa, Oswaldo P. Forattini, Maria Anice Mureb Sallum, Richard C. Wilkinson, and Jeffrey R. Powell, "Short Report: Historical Analysis of a Near Disaster: *Anopheles gambiae* in Brazil," *American Journal of Tropical Medicine and Hygiene*, vol. 78, no. 1 (2008), 176–178.]

had been regionally eliminated.[5] In both Brazil and Egypt, malariologists had laid down the chemical larvicide known as Paris Green, whose insecticidal powers had been part of the antimalaria arsenal since the 1920s.[6]

Another heartening achievement in malaria control – and near eradication – radiated from British Guiana. There, in 1945, the physician and malariologist George Giglioli launched an indoor residual spraying (IRS) program using DDT to control the local vector *An. darlingi*. His approach was so successful that it appeared it might be possible to eradicate locally an indigenous vector and perhaps prevent its reintroduction.[7] By extension, this suggested the possibility of a broader application for vector control in the South American tropics, if the approach could be scaled up. It also suggested the possibility that DDT might be very effective in another tropical context – on the African side of the South Atlantic.

THE TRANSFER OF SYNTHETIC INSECTICIDE, 1945–1950

During the final years of Second World War, American and British military authorities had used synthetic insecticides to spray Allied military barracks and their immediate environs in West Africa. This had proved successful in greatly suppressing malarial infections among the Allied troops stationed there, and, after the war, the spraying expanded beyond the military. The first large-scale use of synthetic insecticides for IRS south of the Sahara began in 1945, in Monrovia, Liberia, and after some initial successes, the malaria program was expanded into

---

[5] The natural insecticide made from chrysanthemum flowers known as pyrethrum was scarce and expensive, but some was held in reserve for use for indoor spraying in the event that larviciding failed to disrupt the breeding of *An. gambiae*. Weekly indoor spraying with pyrethrum was used with good effect in Upper Egypt in the 18,000 houses in the El Badari region. [Aly Tewfik Shousha, "The Eradication of *Anopheles gambiae* from Upper Egypt, 1942–1945," *Bulletin of the World Health Organization*, vol. 1, no. 2 (1948), 309–352; on pyrethrum spraying in El Badari, 326–327.]

[6] The first use of Paris Green was in the 1870s against the Colorado potato beetle. [R. A. Casagrande, "Colorado Potato Beetle: 125 Years of Mismanagement," *Bulletin of the Entomological Society of America*, vol. 33, no. 3 (1987), 144.]

[7] G. Giglioli, "Malaria Control in British Guiana," Bulletin of the World Health Organization, vol. 11 (1954), 849–853; G. Giglioli, *Demerara Doctor: An Early Success against Malaria. The Autobiography of a Self-Taught Physician, George Giglioli (1897–1975)* (London: Smith-Gordon, 2006), 205–218.

the region surrounding Monrovia.[8] A small-scale house-spraying program with DDT began in Southern Rhodesia (now Zimbabwe) the same year, and, in subsequent years, programs of IRS using DDT began in several regions of southern Africa, including South Africa, Swaziland, Bechuanaland (Botswana), and southern Mozambique.[9] In 1947, an experimental IRS program was launched in Freetown, Sierra Leone.[10]

These early IRS programs aimed at the control of malarial disease. As many of these efforts enjoyed success, some of the projects began to focus on localized species eradication. What had worked against invasive species in Brazil and Egypt and against an indigenous species in British Guiana led to hopes for success against indigenous species in tropical Africa.[11]

In the last years of the 1940s, another success in species eradication on the island of Mauritius appeared as a harbinger of future campaigns in the "war on malaria." Even before the arrival in 1948 of a small malaria control team dispatched by the United Kingdom's Colonial Insecticides Committee to attempt species eradication by residual spraying, efforts at malaria control had reduced malaria transmission to virtually nil in the densely populated residential plateau in the middle of the island and the business district of the capital, Port Louis. And from 1949 to 1951, M. A. C. Dowling, a young British physician, led a team that succeeded in eliminating *An. funestus* from the island, completely interrupting malaria transmission and reducing the population of *An. gambiae* by more than 98 percent. In 1951, Dowling tried to move in for the coup de grâce, launching a larvicidal program to eradicate

---

[8] James L. A. Webb, Jr., "The First Large-Scale Use of Synthetic Insecticides to Control Malaria in Tropical Africa: Lessons from Liberia, 1945–1962," *Journal of the History of Medicine and Allied Sciences*, vol. 66, no. 3 (2011), 347–376.

[9] Other IRS programs with DDT began in the 1960s in Namibia and Southern Rhodesia (Zimbabwe). Musawenkosi L. H. Mabaso, Brian Sharp, and Christian Lengeler, "Historical Review of Malarial Control in Southern Africa with Emphasis on the Use of Indoor Residual House-Spraying," *Tropical Medicine and International Health*, vol. 9, no. 8 (2004), 846–856.

[10] The experiment in malaria control in Freetown produced disappointing results. R. Elliott, "Use of DDT as a Residual Insecticide for the Control of Malaria in Freetown," (1947), SJ1, JK1, Sierra Leone, WHO 7.0039, World Health Organization Archives, Geneva.

[11] In the view of Fred Soper of the Rockefeller Foundation, who had directed the campaign against *An. arabiensis* in Brazil, a basic principle was the necessity for an attack on a sufficiently large area so that reinfestation from unworked areas could not pose a problem. [Fred L. Soper, "Species Sanitation as Applied to the Eradication of (A) an Invading or (B) an Indigenous Species," *Proceedings of the Fourth International Congress on Tropical Medicine and Malaria*, vol. 1 (Washington, DC: US Government Printing Office, 1948), 854.]

An. gambiae. Disappointment ensued. Following heavy rainfall in February 1952, *An. gambiae* increased its reproduction in spite of the eradication teams' best efforts. Hopes for species eradication of *An. gambiae* were given up, and future malaria control efforts focused on surveillance and treatment of imported cases.[12]

Even as the Mauritius eradication efforts advanced, malariologists on the African mainland launched some experiments to determine the feasibility of using DDT against the anopheline vectors in rural tropical Africa. The initial results were mixed. In the Kipsigis reserve in western Kenya, 2,500 huts were sprayed with DDT in three cycles in 1946. The experiment reduced deaths in comparison to a control area, drove down parasite rates, and reduced vector density.[13] In March 1949, the Belgian Fonds du Bien-Être Indigène in Ruanda-Urundi, in collaboration with the J. R. Geigy S. A., the Swiss manufacturer of DDT, sprayed a small number of huts in the mountains. The team concluded that IRS would be efficacious in reducing parasite rates, and then scaled up the experiment to cover roughly 20,000 to 23,000 people. Teams of insecticide sprayers doused African huts and anopheline-breeding habitats. Adult mosquito density in the huts declined markedly, but the mosquitoes propagated in their breeding grounds.[14]

Another antimalaria initiative advanced on the highland plateau of Madagascar. There, beginning in 1949, the French launched an ambitious program of IRS and larviciding, combined with weekly chloroquine chemoprophylaxis for children under the age of 15. The program dramatically

---

[12] M. A. C. Dowling, "The Malaria Eradication Scheme in Mauritius," *British Medical Bulletin*, vol. 8, no. 1 (1951), 72–75; M. A. C. Dowling, "Malaria Control in Mauritius," *British Medical Bulletin*, vol. 9 (9 August 1952), 309; M. A. C. Dowling, "Control of Malaria in Mauritius: Eradication of *Anopheles funestus* and *Aedes aegypti*," *Transactions of the Royal Society of Tropical Medicine and Hygiene*, vol. 47, no. 3 (1953), 177–198.

The last indigenous case of malaria occurred in 1965. [Leonard J. Bruce-Chwatt, "Malaria in Mauritius – As Dead as the Dodo," *Bulletin of the New York Academy of Medicine*, vol. 50, no. 10 (November 1974), 1079.]

[13] P. C. C. Garnham, "DDT versus Malaria, Kenya 1946 – Commentary on a Film," in E. E. Sabben-Clare, D. J. Bradley, and K. Kirkwood (eds.), *Health in Tropical Africa during the Colonial Period* (Oxford: Clarendon Press, 1980), 64–65.

[14] WHO7.0038. JKT 1, SJ1. "Compte-rendu concernant l'activité de la Mission d'étude de désinsectisation envoyée au Ruanda-Urundi par le Fonds du Bien-Etre Indigène en collaboration avec la maison J. R. Geigy S. A. Bâle. Février-août 1949," 44–54; J. Jaden, A. Fain, and H. Rupp, "Lutte anti-malarienne étendue en zone rurale au moyen de D.D.T. à Astrida, Ruanda-Urundi," *Institut Royal Colonial Belge, Section des Sciences Naturelles et Médicales, Mémoires*, vol. 21, fasc. 1 (1952), 1–47.

reduced infections, thereby suggesting the possibility of full, if local, erad-ication of malaria.[15]

The World Health Organization (WHO) and the Commission for Technical Cooperation in Africa South of the Sahara jointly convened a Malaria Conference in Equatorial Africa in Kampala, in late 1950. Malariologists from the WHO, many of the European states with colo-nies in tropical Africa (Great Britain, Portugal, France, and Belgium), Liberia, and the United States attended. The participants had the benefit of a report by Dr. F. J. C. Cambournac, a professor at the Lisbon Institute of Tropical Medicine and director of the Institute of Malariology in Portugal. He had been charged by the director-general of the WHO with the preparation of a report on malaria control efforts in equatorial Africa, and, toward this end, he had traveled for more than six months, logging nearly 48,000 miles.[16]

At the Kampala conference, the major policy issue was whether to undertake IRS campaigns in rural African regions of intense malaria trans-mission. It was known that Africans who had survived childhood infec-tions had acquired immunities to malaria and, as a result, suffered less severe bouts of illness. Some were heavily parasitized and remained entirely asymptomatic. The maintenance of acquired immunity was thought to depend on recurrent inoculations with the malarial parasites, and thus the interventions, if successful, might compromise Africans' acquired immunities. If control efforts were subsequently to lapse, the populations that had been protected by the IRS campaigns might suffer "rebound" epidemic malaria, with serious consequences. A partial coun-terargument was that Africans' acquired immunities might well be lost anyway through the movements of rural African laborers to cities, mines, or European-directed plantations. In this view, "economic progress" might involve increases in illness and death for adults with fully functional acquired immunities whose immunological defenses degraded owing to a reduction in infective inoculations.[17]

---

[15] WHO/MAL/150. G. Joncour, "Present Situation in Regard to Malaria Control in Madagascar," 14 November 1955.
[16] WHO/Mal/58. Dr. F. J. C. Cambournac, "Report on Malaria in Equatorial Africa."
[17] WHO/Mal/69. "Report of the Malaria Conference in Equatorial Africa," 22.

During the conference sessions, heated exchanges erupted between the malaria experts. The dispute over IRS was highly contentious because professional opinions differed over whether the high levels of inoculations (and thus the continued challenge by malaria parasites) in regions of heavy endemic transmission produced a fully functional acquired immunity – that is, full protection from malarial sickness in adult populations. Cambournac had put the problem bluntly in his preconference report: "control measures partially carried out or continued for a limited time are dangerous, since the populations of formerly hyperendemic regions will obviously be exposed to the risk of severe epidemics, involving serious consequences."[18] Time-limited or lapsed interventions might well produce sickness and perhaps even deaths in the formerly immune populations.

The experts conceptualized childhood morbidity and mortality as "costs" that were paid to acquire adult and adolescent immunity. Yet, here again, there was fundamental disagreement. How high were the costs of the acquisition of immunity? What was the extent of childhood morbidity and mortality that was attributable to malaria? Professional opinion ranged widely.[19] The British had begun studies in Nigeria, and the preliminary evidence suggested that malaria might account for fully 25 percent of childhood deaths.[20] The extent of childhood medical problems caused or exacerbated by malaria was also unknown. The advocates

---

[18] WHO/Mal/58. Dr. F. J. C. Cambournac, "Report on Malaria in Equatorial Africa," 66.

[19] P. C. C. Garnham, one of the eminent British malariologists in East Africa, conducted postmortem examinations on children in Kisumu, an area of hyperendemic transmission in Kenya. He concluded, in correspondence with his colleague Mr. Paterson, that malaria was rare as a cause of death: "These researches demonstrated the almost complete tolerance rapidly obtained against the parasite in practically all areas and the comparative rarity of Malaria as a cause of death. I have mentioned these observations because, from discussions with many Medical Officers, most appear to hold contrary views on the subject." [Prof. P. C. C. Garnham to Mr. Paterson, 1 June 1942, Native Hospital Kisumu. Correspondence. A.2. No. 11. Papers of Professor Percy Cyril Claude Garnham (1901–1995). Contemporary Medical Archives Centre, Wellcome Institute for the History of Medicine, London.] This position was one that Garnham had held for many years. In the 1930s, Garnham had argued for significant differences in placental malaria between West African and East African populations in regions of hyperendemicity. [P. C. C. Garnham, "Malaria in East Africa," a letter to the editor, *Transactions of the Royal Society of Tropical Medicine and Hygiene*, 24 March 1939.]
   Prof. George Macdonald, the Director of the Ross Institute at the London School of Hygiene and Tropical Medicine, was unimpressed with Garnham's interpretation of the Kisumu data and pointed out flaws in his work. [George Macdonald to P. C. C. Garnham, 5 June 1950. PP/PCG/C22. Contemporary Medical Archives Centre, Wellcome Institute for the History of Medicine, London.]

[20] WHO/Mal/58. Dr. F. J. C. Cambournac, "Report on Malaria in Equatorial Africa," 54.

for greater caution buttressed their arguments with the assumption that childhood mortality costs in areas of heavy endemic transmission were relatively low. The implication – contested by their opponents – was that these putatively low childhood mortality costs might be an acceptable price for fully functional adult immunity.

Two factions formed. One favored malaria intervention using IRS in rural areas using the tools and knowledge at hand. The other favored a more cautious investigation of the consequences of the interruption of acquired immunity. The divisions were bitter. There was agreement that interventions were justified in rural zones of endemic malaria that were subject to epidemic outbreaks. There was no agreement, however, about interventions in rural regions of holoendemic transmission.[21]

At length, the dominant faction at the Kampala conference endorsed a policy proposal to move forward with malaria control as soon as feasible, whatever the degree of endemic transmission. To address the concerns about the potential consequences of the loss of fully functional immunities, the conference report advised that those regions with higher levels of endemic infection would require the establishment of an effective malaria control organization that would be able to intervene with insecticides and drugs, should epidemic malaria erupt after the ending of control projects. It also recommended that the WHO act in an advisory capacity on the malaria control projects in one or more areas in which populations appeared to have a high degree of tolerance to malarial infections.[22]

Important malaria control experiences in African urban zones and their immediate environs were accumulating. Malariologists had scored moderate successes using synthetic larvicides to eliminate mosquito breeding areas within African cities and towns and maintain protective

---

[21] At the Kampala conference, new definitions were agreed on to distinguish between levels of heavy endemic transmission in which there were different percentages of the population with distended spleens. The areas in which the spleen rate in children of 2–10 years of age was constantly more than 50 percent and in which the spleen rate in adults was "high" were to be classified as *hyperendemic*; those areas in which the spleen rate in children of 2–10 years of age was constantly more than 75 percent and in which the spleen rate in adults was "low" were to be classified as *holoendemic*. The "strongest adult tolerance" to malaria was said to be found in holoendemic regions. [*Report on the Malaria Conference in Equatorial Africa*. World Health Organization Technical Report Series, no. 38 (Geneva: World Health Organization, 1951), 45.] Malariologists later discovered regions of heavy endemic malaria transmission in which the spleen rates of the populations did not accord well with these definitional criteria.
[22] WHO/Mal/69. "Report of the Malaria Conference in Equatorial Africa," 41.

belts around urban agglomerations. In Mozambique, for example, Portuguese colonial authorities began an IRS campaign in the African settlements surrounding the port of Lourenço Marques (now, Maputo) in 1946 and extended the program an additional eighteen kilometers into the surrounding territory.[23] House-spraying experiments with DDT had impressively reduced malarial infections, as had house-spraying with benzene hexachloride (BHC).[24] Indeed, these experiences convinced colonial policy-makers who judged that this was the path toward better malaria control in the urban zones of Africa. This was a very different undertaking than the earlier mosquito control efforts that had striven for the elimination of breeding habitat through environmental engineering and the use of larvicides. The use of synthetic insecticides demanded a shift in paradigm: malaria control should target adult mosquitoes, not larvae.[25] A house-spraying project in southwestern Nigeria, using BHC, was already in progress. Its aim was to investigate the practicality of using IRS alone to create a malaria-free "island" in rural tropical Africa, in an extension of the practice of creating protective belts around urban agglomerations. The center of the island was the town of Ilaro with 12,000 inhabitants, surrounded by secondary forest.[26]

Three lines of argument provided the economic rationale for IRS intervention in rural Africa. First, malaria imposed high economic costs. Second, the lifting of the malarial burden would be necessary for economic growth and development. And third, IRS would be the least expensive and thus, in the acutely resource-scarce context of the postwar years, the only practical method of control.[27] Empirical investigations were still in their

---

[23] Alberto Soeiro, Mário Pereira, and Artur Pereira, "A Luta Anti-Malárica em Lourenço Marques," *Anais do Instituto de Medecina Tropical*, vol. 13, no. 4 (1956), 635–669.

[24] WHO/Mal/58. Dr. F. J. C. Cambournac, "Report on Malaria in Equatorial Africa," 21–26.

[25] WHO/Mal/58. Dr. F. J. C. Cambournac, "Report on Malaria in Equatorial Africa," 32.

[26] The project had been suggested by the WHO Expert Committee on Malaria in 1948. See WHO/MAL/40. L. J. Bruce-Chwatt et al., "The Ilaro Experimental Vector Species Eradication Scheme by Residual Insecticide Spraying (First Progress Report)," 5 May 1950; L. J. Bruce-Chwatt, H. Archibald, R. Elliott, R. A. Fitz-John, and I. A. Balogus, "Ilaro Experimental Malaria Control Scheme: Report on Four Years' Results," *Fifth International Congress on Tropical Medicine and Malaria*, vol. 2 *Communications* (Istanbul, 1953), 54–66.

[27] For a general statement of the issues, see G. Macdonald, "The Economic Importance of Malaria in Africa," 24 October 1950, WHO/MAL/60.

Health gains from malaria interventions were evident in areas where the malaria burden was seasonal, the degree of acquired immunity was not robust, the average adult received relatively few inoculations per season, and the inoculations produced sickness. In this paper, Macdonald also attacked the views of malariologists who held that adult

early stages, but this rationale was bolstered by the experiences with malaria control in the Transvaal, where South African authorities reported an improvement in overall "native" health and fewer workdays lost to sickness.[28] The lesson drawn was that malaria control could be a profound stimulus to economic growth.

At Kampala, the experts agreed, given the state of knowledge at the time, on the impossibility of recommending any standard protocol for malaria control for rural tropical Africa. At mid-century, the core empirical questions were yet to be answered. Would it be possible to interrupt the transmission of malaria in rural tropical Africa through the use of the new synthetic insecticides? If so, which insecticides should be used, in what dosages and treatment cycles, at what financial costs, and in which zones? As the final report stated, "The diversity of features of this continent is such that each project should be specially designed to meet the particular situation and to deal with it by the most satisfactory and economical ways."[29]

IN THE AFTERMATH OF THE KAMPALA CONFERENCE

In the early 1950s, the medical community moved closer to a consensus on the high costs of childhood mortality. The estimate of 25 percent of childhood mortality directly attributable to malaria, based on studies at Ilaro, came to be more widely accepted, and thus, for those who accepted this estimate, one of the reasons for caution in malaria intervention dissipated. By virtue of the good that could be conveyed to those in the early years of life through the prevention of malaria transmission, the concern over the harm that might be done to adults in areas of heavy transmission whose acquired immunities had been compromised through lapsed malaria interventions went to the back burner. With enthusiasm for the prospects for full success, the experts left the ethical ramifications of lapsed malaria interventions unexplored.[30]

populations in "hyperendemic" African regions had achieved a perfect balance with the malarial parasites.

[28] Randall Packard, "'Malaria Blocks Development' Revisited: The Role of Disease in the History of Agricultural Development in the Eastern and Northern Transvaal Lowveld, 1890–1960," *Journal of Southern African Studies*, vol. 27, no. 3 (2001), 591–612.

[29] WHO/Mal/69. "Report of the Malaria Conference in Equatorial Africa," 46.

[30] The issue of acquired immunities to falciparum malaria had salience principally in tropical Africa. It was not a central issue in the broader global campaign to eradicate malaria (1955–1969) because on no other subcontinental region was falciparum transmission maintained at such high levels.

Malariologists expected that new technical challenges would arise in different African ecological settings. In preparation for the Kampala conference, Cambournac had compiled a list of institutions concerned with malaria interventions and research, and this provided a rough overview of the interventions in progress. Following the Kampala conference, the role of WHO malaria experts was as technical advisors on projects that would be supported with United Nations Children's Fund (UNICEF) monies to investigate the possibility of moving from malaria control to the cessation of malaria transmission.

In 1955, the governing body of the WHO, the World Health Assembly, voted in favor of a program for the global eradication of malaria. The program would grow in size to become the largest undertaking to date of the WHO and the first-ever attempt to eradicate a disease. Across the globe, national malaria eradication programs began their work. In tropical Africa, the hope was that pilot malaria eradication projects would be able to determine the most cost-effective applications of the new synthetic insecticides and that these insecticides would be able fully to interrupt malaria transmission (Figure 3.1). If the best and least expensive practices could be determined, it might be possible to scale up these pilot projects. If so, tropical African colonies and states might undertake full-scale eradication programs similar to those unfolding on other continents burdened with malaria.

THE WHO PROJECT SITES

The WHO pilot projects were launched in forest, savanna, sahelian, coastal, and highland zones in tropical Africa (see Map 3.1). One of the pilot projects radiated out from the city of Yaoundé in southern Cameroun in an effort to create a larger malaria-free zone that extended deep into the surrounding rural hinterland. The focus of the other pilot projects, however, was within rural zones. Long experience with urban and enclave malaria interventions suggested, at a minimum, that malaria infections could be dramatically reduced in these settings, given a sufficiently large outlay of funds. In rural areas – beyond the European farms and plantations – the charge was different. Where there was no prospect of securing funding for ongoing rural projects, malariologists focused on a permanent solution to the malaria problem. Would it be possible to fully interrupt transmission at an affordable cost?

The idea of eradication was based on two premises. The first was that if transmission could be interrupted, it would be possible to proceed to

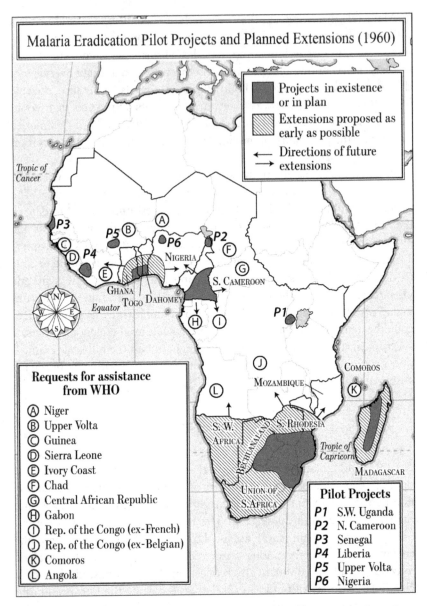

Malaria Eradication Pilot Projects and Planned Extensions (1960)

Projects in existence
or in plan

Extensions proposed as
early as possible

← Directions of future
→ extensions

Tropic of Cancer

P3
P5 Ⓑ   Ⓐ
Ⓒ   *P6*   *P2*
Ⓓ *P4*   NIGERIA   Ⓕ
Ⓔ   Ⓖ
            S. CAMEROON
GHANA
Equator TOGO DAHOMEY
            Ⓗ Ⓘ   *P1*

            Ⓙ   COMOROS
        MOZAMBIQUE
Ⓛ   Ⓚ

**Requests for assistance
from WHO**

Ⓐ Niger
Ⓑ Upper Volta
Ⓒ Guinea
Ⓓ Sierra Leone
Ⓔ Ivory Coast
Ⓕ Chad
Ⓖ Central African Republic
Ⓗ Gabon
Ⓘ Rep. of the Congo (ex-French)
Ⓙ Rep. of the Congo (ex-Belgian)
Ⓚ Comoros
Ⓛ Angola

S. W.
AFRICA   S. RHODESIA
          *Tropic of
          Capricorn*
                  MADAGASCAR
UNION OF
S. AFRICA

Pilot Projects

P1	S.W. Uganda
P2	N. Cameroon
P3	Senegal
P4	Liberia
P5	Upper Volta
P6	Nigeria

MAP 3.1. Malaria Eradication Pilot Projects and Planned Extensions (1960)
Adapted from the World Health Organization (WHO) Regional Office for Africa,
Afro Malaria Yearbook No. 2 (Geneva: WHO, 1960).

eradication. The absence of local transmission would equate to the local disappearance of the disease, and the protocols for successful eradication, once established, could eventually be scaled up over entire regions. This did not take account of the problem of latent asymptomatic infections. The second premise was that the costs of the local interruption of transmission, even if substantial, would involve a single time-limited expenditure of funds. There was, at the time, no appreciation of the fact that the costs of surveillance after the interruption of transmission could dwarf initial expenditures.

The hopes for the complete interruption of malaria transmission by killing adult mosquitoes sailed forward on the winds of optimism about the powers of the new synthetic insecticides. Whereas the success of the antimosquito measures of the earlier twentieth century had rested principally on killing mosquito larva in situ and/or destroying mosquito habitat, the new generation of synthetic insecticides trumped the older on two counts. First, the synthetic insecticides were far less expensive. This meant that a given budget could be used to reach many more people. Second, at least some of the new insecticides, when sprayed on buildings, left behind long-acting residues. This raised hopes that per unit spraying costs would be dramatically lower. The approach was undergirded by an elegant mathematical model of malarial dynamics developed by George MacDonald at the London School of Hygiene and Tropical Medicine that emphasized the disruption of malaria transmission that could be accomplished by killing adult female anophelines with synthetic insecticides.[31]

In practice, the application of synthetic insecticides in tropical Africa was far from straightforward. The insecticides interacted with house materials in unpredictable ways. Some modes of house construction required a great deal more insecticide than others, and on some house materials, emulsion sprays worked better than wettable powders. Rainy seasons wreaked havoc on indoor residual sprays and thus the cycle of sprayings – once, twice, thrice, or even twelve times a year – had to be worked out locally on an empirical basis.

Other problems, however, proved more or less intractable. In Liberia, for example, the eradication pilot project managers assumed that they would spray the houses in all of the villages in the project zones. They did not take account of the fact that the villagers spent part of the

---

[31] George MacDonald, *The Epidemiology and Control of Malaria* (London: Oxford University Press, 1957).

agricultural season near their fields, living in seasonal shelters that had roofs but no walls.[32]

THE ENTOMOLOGICAL LABYRINTH

The effective application of insecticides also depended on an understanding of the behavior of the African mosquito vectors. At the time, much was yet unknown, and the experts at the 1950 Kampala conference were agreed that basic research on the principal African vectors was essential. Their emphasis on the need for local entomological investigation as a basic foundation of malaria control was very much in line with the development of malariology elsewhere. It was part of what today would be called "best practice." In tropical Africa, local entomological studies proved greatly complex. One key issue was the ecological range of *An. gambiae*. Good progress was made toward a fuller appreciation of the complex of related species, with different behaviors and genetic susceptibilities to insecticides.[33] Yet as researchers on the *An. gambiae* complex made important advances and drew important distinctions, the role of entomology in the antimalaria projects was downgraded. As the killing powers of synthetic insecticides in tropical Africa were brought to bear, research on mosquitoes seemed less important: if the insecticides worked against all vector mosquitoes, what was the point of spending resources on understanding microvariations in feeding, breeding, alighting, or other bionomic matters? A gulf began to open up between the entomologists and the project managers whose understanding of mosquito species was rudimentary at best.

Some basic mosquito behaviors appeared to be well enough understood to permit the pilot projects to move forward. A widely shared belief was that both *An. gambiae* and *An. funestus* were largely endophagic; that is, that the female took her blood meal indoors. Indeed, this was the foundational rationale for IRS: when the female mosquito alighted on a sprayed surface, either before or after she took her blood meal, she would pick up enough insecticide to cause her death. Confidence in the indoor-resting, or endophilic, behavior of *An. gambiae* and *An. funestus* was strong. The behaviors of the other African anopheline vectors were less certain but seemed of only minor importance. It did not

[32] Webb, "First Large-Scale Use," 360–361.
[33] M. H. Holstein, *Biology of Anopheles gambiae. Research in French West Africa.* World Health Organization monograph no. 9 (Geneva: WHO, 1954).

initially occur to the researchers that the two principal African vectors might have a range of specialized feeding and resting behaviors that could be influenced by IRS.

THE MIXED RECORD OF SYNTHETIC INSECTICIDES

In line with the recommendations of the Kampala conference and those of the Colonial Insecticides Committee in the United Kingdom, the malaria control project managers experimented with a number of different synthetic pesticides. DDT and lindane (gamma-hexachlorocyclohexane, also known as gammexane or HCH)[34] had been used to control malaria in urban settings in a very minor role during the final years of the war and in a larger role beginning in 1945, at the transition from the use of the older generation of larvicides such as Paris Green and malariol.

The initial postwar experience with DDT in tropical Africa was mixed. In Monrovia, Liberia, for example, beginning in 1945, the Americans oversaw the spraying of DDT for both IRS and larvicidal purposes throughout the city and its surroundings. DDT spraying had little direct killing or residual effect because the house materials were sorptive. Houses had to be sprayed frequently, and the costs were prohibitive.[35] In Freetown, Sierra Leone, the use of DDT also produced disappointing results.[36] The overall judgment of the Colonial Insecticides Committee in 1947 was negative: "it appears that in its present form at least D.D.T. in Kerosene applied as a residual insecticide in West African village houses may not be of very great value in reducing the numbers and infectivity of Anopheles."[37] Greater success seemed to be promised by a shift to a new chlorinated hydrocarbon, first produced in 1948, known as dieldrin (DLD).

---

[34] In the malariological literature of the era, BHC was sometimes also referred to as gammexane.

[35] Webb, "First Large-Scale Use," 354–355.

[36] As F. Maclagan, acting director of medical services, Medical Department, Freetown, put it: "The treatment of Freetown with D.D.T. solution has not prevented mosquito nuisance, and has had no measurable effect on room density indices. As a malaria control measure no form of residual insecticide has so far been shown to be effective under West African conditions." [NAUK, CO/554/153/1, F. Maclagan, "Use of D.D.T. as a Residual Insecticide for the Control of Malaria in Freetown"]

[37] NAUK, CO 911/1. Colonial Pesticides Committee, "Summary of Experiments on the Effects of House Spraying with Pyrethrum and with D.D.T. in Kerosene on *A. gambiae* and *A. melas* in West Africa." Colonial Medical Research Committee, CIC (47) 3 C.M.R. (46) 72, 20th December 1946.

This was a common pattern throughout the West African projects: an experimental turn toward dieldrin, which had a long residual action like DDT, and, in some cases, toward benzene hexachloride (BHC). (HCH had a very weak residual action.) Both DLD and BHC produced a greater immediate mosquito kill rate than did DDT.[38] Yet mosquito resistance to DLD (which conveyed a cross-resistance to HCH) developed rapidly – often within a year or so of extensive use. Resistance was first noted in northwestern Nigeria in 1956, and, by the early 1960s, resistance had spread over a vast area of West Africa, from the Gambia and Mali to Congo and Northern Cameroon. In 1961, cross-resistance between BHC and DLD emerged in northern Cameroon, and for the first time in tropical Africa, also in northern Cameroon, researchers documented vector resistance to DDT.[39] In the following years, experts suspected that DDT resistance had also emerged in Senegal and in Congo, although this seemed to be of little practical significance; in many West African projects, the use of DDT had not been able to interrupt the transmission of malaria.[40] These West African experiences with synthetic insecticides differed from those in East Africa. There, *An. gambiae* and the other malaria vectors did not develop resistance to either DLD or BHC. The absence of this constraint meant that there was less need for experimentation. The pilot project at Kigezi in Uganda used DDT exclusively; the malaria control project at

---

[38] Dieldrin also exacted a human cost: on some malaria control projects, the spraymen suffered dieldrin poisoning. The problem was documented as early as 1955 in Nigeria; the use of dieldrin continued for several years across tropical Africa. [Wayland J. Hayes, Jr., "Dieldrin Poisoning in Man," *Public Health Reports*, vol. 72, no. 12 (1957), 1087–1091. The Nigerian experience was documented in J. Haworth, "Observations on the Possible Toxic Effects of Dieldrin," WHO/Insecticides/60, 1955, cited by Hayes, "Dieldrin Poisoning," 1088; see also WHO/MAL/215, Wayland J. Hayes, Jr., "Report on the Toxicity of Dieldrin to Man," 5 January 1959.] Studies at the malaria control project at Pare-Taveta in Tanganyika, where spraymen adhered closely to guidelines to limit contamination, found no evidence of clinical symptoms of dieldrin poisoning. [T. E. Fletcher, J. M. Press, and D. Bagster Wilson, "Exposure of Spray-men to Dieldrin in Residual Spraying," *Bulletin of the World Health Organization*, vol. 20, no. 1 (1959), 15–25.]

[39] WHO/MAL/323. Ph. Cavalié and J. Mouchet, "The Experimental Malaria Eradication Campaign in the North of the Republic of Cameroon. II. Anti-malaria Operations and Their Results," 8 December 1961, 21.

[40] J. Hamon and J. Mouchet, "La résistance aux insecticides chez les insects d'importance médicale. Méthodes d'étude et situation en Afrique au sud du Sahara," *Médecine tropicale*, vol. 21, no. 5 (1961), 565–596; J. Mouchet and J. Hamon, "Les problèmes techniques de l'éradication du paludisme en Afrique," *Cahiers O.R.S.T.O.M.*, Série Entomologie Médicale, vol. 33 (1963), 39–48; J. Coz and J. Hamon, "Importance pratique de la résistance aux insecticides en Afrique au sud du Sahara pour l'éradication du paludisme dans ce continent," *Cahiers O.R.S.T.O.M.*, Série Entomologie Médicale, no. 1 (1963), 77–83.

Pare-Taveta on the Kenya/Tanzanian border never used DDT.[41] These West and East African experiences differed, in turn, from those in southern Africa. There, the vectors were less efficient, the house materials were less problematic for spraying on insecticides, malaria transmission was markedly seasonal, and the levels of endemicity were low. The malaria control services based their successful programs on the indoor spraying of houses with BHC, as well as with DDT.[42]

ANTIMALARIAL DRUGS AND THE PILOT PROJECTS

By the mid 1950s, as evidence began to accumulate from the first cluster of pilot projects that IRS alone would not be able to interrupt transmission, malariologists designed the second cluster of projects either with a chemoprophylactic or chemotherapeutic component or both.[43] At a WHO technical meeting on African malaria held in Brazzaville in 1957, malaria experts unanimously recommended the initiation of large-scale experiments with the mass administration of antimalarials. The recommendation was to employ different drugs and dosage schedules to determine the efficacy of the interventions.[44]

The mass administration of antimalarial drugs had a long and checkered history into the mid-twentieth century. The Italians had undertaken the first national mass drug administration program, with mixed success. In a mixed malarial environment of vivax, falciparum, and malariae infections, the mass administration of quinine had dramatically reduced malarial deaths, but not morbidity.[45]

[41] WHO/MAL/394. J. Mouchet and J. Hamon, "Difficulties in Malaria Eradication Campaigns Due to the Behaviour of the Vectors," 16 May 1963, 7; WHO/MAL/336. J. Hamon, "Insecticide-Resistance in Major Vectors of Malaria, and Its Operational Significance," 22 March 1962, 12.
[42] WHO AFRO/MAL/2. [n. a.], "Malaria in the African Region. A Review," 20 August 1958, 9.
   Later, DDT resistance in the Transvaal and DDT, DLD, and HCH resistance in Swaziland emerged. See the WHO map, "Countries with Insecticide Resistance in Anopheles Mosquitoes of Particular Importance," held by the WHO archives in Geneva. [Undated, it has no formal finding code and is filed with WHO disease maps.]
[43] WHO/MAL/137. Max J. Miller, "Chemotherapy in Malaria Control," 20 September 1955; WHO/MAL/147. I.H. Vincke, "Place of Chemotherapy in Modern Malaria Control Programs," 27 October 1955; WHO/MAL/175. L.J. Bruce-Chwatt, "Chemotherapy in Relation to Possibilities of Malaria Eradication in Tropical Africa," 21 May 1956.
[44] AFR/MAL/39. M.A.C. Dowling, "The Use of Mass Drug Administration in Malaria Projects in the African Region," [n. d.; circa 1961], 1.
[45] Frank M. Snowden, *The Conquest of Malaria: Italy*, 53–114.

In tropical Africa before the Second World War, there had been no comparable experience with mass drug administration of quinine. The British and French colonial powers had set up cinchona plantations during the interwar years, but the quantities of cinchona alkaloids produced had been small. Some Africans, particularly those living in urban areas, acquired quinine through post office sales of individual doses, but the number of individuals who availed themselves of this chemical therapy was relatively small. From a public health point of view, the scant local supplies and the high cost of quinine on the international market had excluded the option of mass campaigns. In the 1930s, the Americans had experimented on African workers in Liberia with plasmochin, which offered the prospect for a reduction in transmission through the destruction of gametocytes, but the plasmochin experiments had seemed impracticable and had not led to broader programs of mass drug administration.

In the postwar period, however, the availability of synthetic drugs opened up new possibilities for malaria interventions. The synthetic drugs pyrimethamine and chloroquine seemed to have fewer side effects than quinine.[46] Both could serve either as a malaria prophylaxis or a cure. As the price of the synthetic drugs dropped, their sheer inexpensiveness allowed malariologists to consider deploying the drugs in new roles. They might limit the damage from outbreaks of epidemic malaria in highland areas in which African populations had little or no immunity, interrupt transmission before or during an IRS campaign, protect the young in the absence of other efforts to control malaria, and/or reduce malaria during

---

[46] As M. Robert, M. le Médecin Général Inspecteur, Directeur Général de la Santé Publique en A. O. F., put it: "Certains essais de chimio-prophylaxie de mass par la quinine et même dans certains cas par les synthétiques, ont fait apparaître la fièvre bilieuse hémoglobinurique avec une grande fréquence chez les africains, alors que cetter affection était extrêmement rare chex eux avant l'introduction des anti-malariques et était réservée à l'européen non immunisé par les infections de l'enfance et soumis à une prophylaxie quinuinique mal appliquée....

"Il est remarquable, et ceci est démontré par les statistiques, comme par l'expérience des médecins des hôpitaux d'A.O.F., que la fièvre bilieuse hémoglobinurique est en voie de disparition depuis l'utilisation de la chimio-prophylaxie individuelle des produits synthéthiques.

"Appliquer à l'africain une chimio-prophylaxie quininque généralisée serait, dans les conditions actuelles, aboutir, non à l'éradication du paludisme – puisque les conditions de transmission persisteraient – mais à une dimunition dangereuse de son remarkable pouvoir de résistance vis-à-vis des complications sévères du paludisme." [IMTSSA, Box 232. Dossier Antipaludiques. M. Robert, M. le Médecin Général Inspecteur, Directeur Général de la Santé Publique en A.O.F., "Note au sujet de: La Quinine dans la lutte anti-palustre en A.O.F.," 3.]

the transmission season, whether or not other control efforts were ongoing. If the insecticides alone were capable of greatly reducing but not completely interrupting transmission, the drugs might be able to clean up the human reservoir of parasites and perhaps reach the goal of zero transmission. Another possibility was that the drugs might be used for regular, ongoing mass chemoprophylaxis.[47]

A major challenge was how to get drugs to rural populations within a project zone. One option was mixing antimalarial medicines into sodium chloride, on the theory that everybody consumed salt. Moderately large-scale distributions of chloroquine-medicated salt were introduced into a zone of 30,000 people in northern Ghana and into communities of laborers with a total population of more than 23,000 who worked on two sugar estates in Uganda. Both programs ran into insurmountable difficulties, including the rejection (or nonuse) of the medicated salt.[48] A trial in Tanzania, in a region in which the supply of salt could be completely controlled, in conjunction with a successful health propaganda campaign, produced a short-term medical success.[49]

In Bobo-Dioulasso in Upper Volta (now Burkina Faso) and at Bernin Kebbi in northern Nigeria, project managers oversaw the direct distribution of antimalarial tablets to Africans in the project zones. In Uganda and in northern Cameroon, the project authorities tried a monitored distribution of a single-dose of antimalarial drug during the spraying cycle, and this approach succeeded in further reducing parasite prevalence.

---

[47] The French had a different view of the prospects for mass antimalarial prophylaxis than did the British. In 1949, the French launched an extensive program of malaria control on the island of Madagascar that used mass chemoprophylaxis, and this interest was extended to their antimalaria projects on the mainland. The French medical legacy continued after independence: Cameroon and Senegal developed national antimalaria chemoprophylaxis programs. [A. B. G. Laing, "The Impact of Malaria Chemoprophylaxis in Africa with Special Reference to Madagascar, Cameroon, and Senegal," *Bulletin of the World Health Organization*, vol. 62, supplement (1984), 41–48.]

The British never developed such programs in their African colonies, and neither did any of the independent African states that gained their independence from the British. The British view was that regular prophylaxis did not make much sense in tropical Africa because the high rate of malaria transmission (in conjunction with a concern about compromising the immunological status of Africans) meant that a regime of prophylaxis would demand high levels of compliance, and this was deemed unachievable.

[48] S. A. Hall and N. E. Wilks, "A Trial of Chloroquine-Medicated Salt for Malaria Suppression in Uganda," *American Journal of Tropical Medicine and Hygiene*, vol. 16, no. 4 (1967), 429–442; WHO Archives, Geneva, WHO7.0017, SJ 5, JKT 1, Ghana, [n. a.], "Assessment Report on the Ghana-18 Medicated Salt Pilot Project," 2.

[49] D. F. Clyde, "Suppression of Malaria in Tanzania with the Use of Medicated Salt," *Bulletin of the World Health Organization*, vol. 35, no. 6 (1966), 962–968.

Monitored distribution, however, proved too costly to be scaled up. An alternate approach was via unmonitored direct distribution – which meant providing drugs to village heads or other local authorities who, in turn, distributed them. In Madagascar, Ghana, and Senegal, there were programs of unmonitored direct distribution of antimalarials for long-term prophylaxis. Costs were lower, but the effectiveness of distribution diminished quickly, and the programs ran the risk of inadvertent overdosing.

Researchers judged the overall results of the chemotherapeutic interventions to be unimpressive. In monitored distribution schemes in Upper Volta, northern Cameroon, Ghana, and northern Nigeria, pyrimethamine was initially highly efficacious, but it selected for resistance in the falciparum parasite within a few months. Chloroquine alone or in combination with primaquine, which killed falciparum gametocytes, also cleared infections, but the prospects for long-term prophylaxis were poor. The major impediment – nearly insuperable – was the establishment of a regular rhythm of distribution and use. Moreover, the utility of mass drug distribution schemes was called into question by their apparent inability to achieve project goals. In combination with IRS, antimalarial drugs could drive rates of infection extremely low, but not to the point of fully interrupting transmission.[50] See Figures 3.1 through 3.4.

THE LOSS OF ACQUIRED IMMUNITIES AND EPIDEMIC "REBOUND" MALARIA

In the aftermath of the lapsed pilot projects, malaria transmission increased. L. J. Bruce-Chwatt, one of the leading malariologists from the United Kingdom who had strongly advocated for insecticide spraying in rural Africa at the Kampala Conference, found the evidence about resurgent

---

[50] J. Hamon, J. Mouchet, and G. Chauvet, "Bilan de quatorze années de lutte contre le paludisme dans les pays francophones d'Afrique tropicale et à Madagascar. Considérations sur la persistance de la transmission et perspectives d'avenir," *Bulletin de la Société de pathologie exotique*, t. 56, no. 5 (septembre–octobre 1963), 945–946.

On the islands of Zanzibar and Pemba, the combination of IRS with synthetic insecticides and the distribution of chloroquine was highly successful in driving the infection rates to very low levels. The relatively small surface areas of the two islands facilitated these successes. By 1966, there were few infections to treat. Parasitized workers from the mainland, however, came to the islands seeking seasonal work, and when malaria control loosened, malaria transmission was re-established. For details, see David F. Clyde, *Malaria in Tanzania* (London: Oxford University Press, 1967).

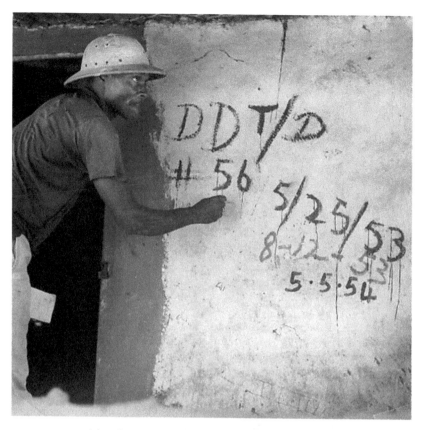

FIGURE 3.1. After the spraying is completed in any house the foreman records the date of spraying on the wall. Photograph by P. Palmer. WHO Photo 1991, PRINT-AFRO-MALARIA. WHO Copyright, used by permission.

malaria highly mixed and difficult to interpret.[51] Some clinical studies advanced evidence that individuals who were reinfected with malaria parasites after having been resident in a malaria eradication pilot project zone might be free of disease symptoms. Was the asymptomatism merely evidence that the interventions had not continued long enough to cause a fuller

[51] L. J. Bruce-Chwatt investigated the state of knowledge of this issue in his 1962 report "A Longitudinal Survey of Natural Malaria Infection in a Group of West African Adults," 17 December 1962, WHO/MAL/369. This work was also published as "A Longitudinal Survey of Natural Malaria Infection in a Group of West African Adults. I," *West African Medical Journal*, vol. 12 (1963), 141–173 and "A Longitudinal Survey of Natural Malaria Infection in a Group of West African Adults. II," *West African Medical Journal*, vol. 12 (1963), 199–217.

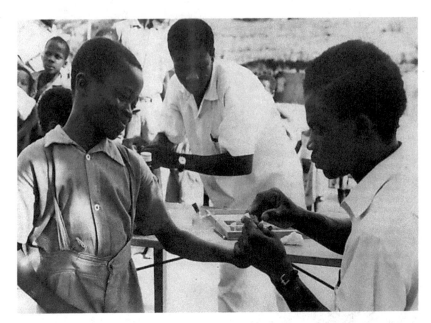

FIGURE 3.2. Laboratory technicians collect blood specimens from school children in a survey to determine the incidence of malaria in the town of Ho. Photographer unknown. WHO Photo 11761, PRINT-AFRO-MALARIA. WHO Copyright, used by permission.

degradation of the individual's immune status? Or was the asymptomatism an indication that the degradation was not a serious problem?

Other studies indicated that the resurgence of malaria took epidemic form with severe consequences. In the aftermath of the pilot project near Yaoundé, the resurgence produced acute malaria at levels that had only exceptionally been previously recorded.[52] In the aftermath of the pilot project in the Kpain region of central Liberia, epidemic malaria struck adults as well as children in the once protected communities.[53] At Pare-Taveta, malaria transmission was re-established, but the incidence of mortality and morbidity was lower than what the experts had anticipated, probably owing to the availability of inexpensive antimalarial drugs and extensive self-medication.[54]

[52] WHO/MAL/369. Bruce-Chwatt, "A Longitudinal Survey," 62.
[53] Webb, "First Large-Scale Use," 366.
[54] C. C. Draper, J. L. M. Lelijveld, Y. G. Matola, and G. B. White, "Malaria in the Pare Area of Tanzania. IV. Malaria in the Human Population 11 Years after the Suspension of Residual Insecticide Spraying, with Special Reference to the Serological Findings,"

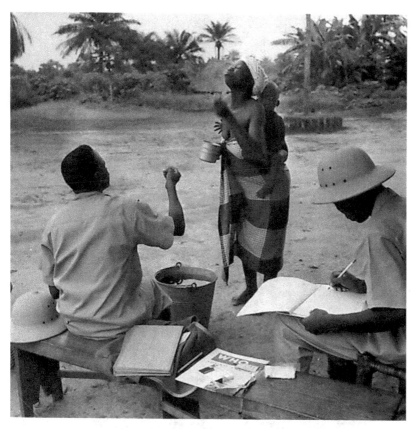

FIGURE 3.3. In the village of Gehtar, Liberia, anti-malaria tablets are distributed which children and grown-ups swallow with enthusiasm. Photograph by Paul Almasy. WHO Photo 7141, ARCO 12, PRINT-AFRO-MALARIA. WHO Copyright, used by permission.

The situation was complex and difficult to conceptualize because when "rebound" epidemic malaria struck, the disease consequences went largely unmeasured. Although the Kampala conference had recommended that malaria control services be established to allow for effective intervention in the case of rebound malaria, this recommendation had not been implemented. The malaria control projects had not been charged to create a malaria service or any other type of public health infrastructure, and the

Transactions of the Royal Society of Tropical Medicine and Hygiene, vol. 66, no. 6 (1972), 905–912.

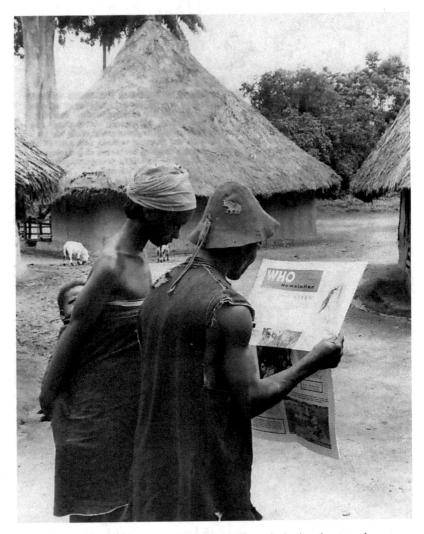

FIGURE 3.4. A mobile team has to march through the brush to reach a group of villages deep in the jungle. The team's sanitary inspector had brought along some WHO publications on malaria. Photograph by Paul Almasy. WHO Photo 7144, ARCO 12, PRINT-AFRO-MALARIA. WHO Copyright, used by permission.

institutional capacities for medical surveillance in tropical Africa in the 1950s and early 1960s were rudimentary at best.

The lack of medical surveillance allowed for the ethical dimensions of the lapsed control projects to be ignored. Some evidence – such as the spike in adult spleen rates that was noted in the aftermath of the closure of a pilot project in Liberia – indicated that a part of the malarial burden had been shifted to age cohorts that had previously been protected by their acquired immunities.[55]

THE LESSONS OF THE MALARIA CONTROL AND ERADICATION PROJECTS

In the early 1960s, after years of effort that had protected millions of Africans, the WHO malariologists closed down the malaria eradication pilot projects. They had accumulated a wealth of practical experience across tropical Africa. They had analyzed data on morbidity and mortality, mosquitoes, parasites, spleen rates, fevers, and insecticides, and they had grappled with the organizational challenges of indoor residual house-spraying and the distribution of antimalarial drugs. The malariologists had sought to develop eradication protocols that, subject to local conditions, could be used across the continent.

The malariologists had been little attuned to the African social universes in whose midst their antimalaria projects unfolded, and the projects advanced largely without input from communities in the project zones. The cultural gulf remained fundamentally unbridged. Project workers discovered that many Africans were not interested in ingesting salt laced with antimalarial drugs and that many were unwilling to take regular doses of prophylactic pills. Many Africans became fatigued with the household disruptions that accompanied the cycles of IRS, and after the sprayed insecticides stopped working against household bugs and vermin, some closed their doors to the spray teams.

The malariologists were also unprepared for the extent of the movement of people between a project zone and its surrounding region. The project zones had been established as territorial blocs, with treated areas adjoining untreated zones that served to provide baseline data. These population movements confounded the malariologists' work because parasitized individuals from unsprayed areas reignited malarial infections in villages where transmission had been reduced to near zero. The problem became complicated further when people moved across state boundaries.[56]

---

[55] Webb, "First Large-Scale Use," 366.
[56] The outstanding scholar of African migration and malaria was R. Mansell Prothero, who produced a series of WHO reports culminating in his book *Migrants and Malaria* (London: Longman, 1965).

The issue of migration had daunting implications. It meant that malarial infections could be introduced and exchanged across virtually the entirety of sub-Saharan Africa.[57] Any antimalaria campaign that aimed at zero transmission would require the cooperation of the governments in the adjoining states. This was a tremendous challenge because the newly independent governments (and the central governments of Liberia and Ethiopia) had little effective reach into large parts of their state territories. And if national governments were weak, a successful antimalaria campaign would have to engage the energies and interests of indigenous political authorities. This was a large charge because the cultural gaps in perception about the significance of malaria were great.

The aborted malaria eradication campaign had been driven by the insights and assumptions of Western bioscience. Western perceptions of the seriousness of malaria were honed by knowledge about the vulnerability of nonimmunes in tropical Africa, economic arguments about the loss of worker productivity, and growing evidence that malaria killed many African children and wreaked havoc with the lives of some who survived. African perceptions were very different. Africans thought about the serious complications of malaria for children using very different cosmological frameworks from those of the Western-trained biomedical workers.[58] Moreover, most Africans thought of these childhood afflictions as quite distinct from the fevers and flu-like symptoms experienced by Africans who had achieved robust levels of acquired immunity. For African adults, malaria was largely perceived as an annoyance, an unpleasant reality of life like the seasonal flu, rather than a vital problem to be tackled with scarce resources. At independence, most African states declined to take up the "pre-eradication" programs – in essence, malaria control programs that would be developed to build capacity – recommended by the WHO.

On the technical side, the antimalaria projects demonstrated that indoor spraying with residual insecticides and the use of antimalarial drugs to prevent or to clear infections at the population level could greatly reduce the transmission of malaria but could not reduce the levels to zero. One lesson drawn from the projects was that malaria *eradication* in tropical Africa was not feasible, given the extant tools, resources, and constraints. The corollary was that malaria *control* was feasible and that it might be achieved if Africans prioritized malaria as a critically important health

---

[57] Sub-Saharan falciparum infections were unable to gain a footing in Europe owing to the lack of susceptibility of the Mediterranean vectors to the African genotypes.

[58] See, for example, Alma Gottlieb, *The Afterlife Is Where We Come From.*

issue. The issue of the financial sustainability of long-term malaria control remained moot. Except in a few areas of southern Africa, within states governed by Europeans, long-term programs were not put in place.

The control and eradication projects also pointed toward the conclusion that residual insecticides could not be used indefinitely to control malaria. All of the insecticides – HCH, BHC, DLD, and to a lesser extent DDT – had selected for vector resistance. The antimalarial drugs appeared to operate similarly in a parallel domain. The mass use of the drug pyrimethamine had quickly selected for parasite resistance, and it seemed that other antimalarials might eventually do the same. Although in 1965 widespread falciparum resistance to chloroquine in tropical Africa lay some years in the future, some prescient malariologists anticipated its emergence.

The pilot malaria eradication projects, however, had also bequeathed a key cautionary lesson that was not assimilated. It was the same one that had been taught at Freetown in the aftermath of the Second World War. The failed pilot projects had produced untoward malarial dynamics in their wakes. Severe morbidity and an increased incidence of mortality had been inflicted on those age cohorts whose acquired immunities had been lost during the era of malaria control. The extent and the ethical dimensions of this medical crisis for African adolescents, parents, and grandparents in the project zones went unexplored.

4

Positive Turbulence

The efforts to control malaria in tropical Africa met with resistance in the world of politics as well as in the realms of parasites and mosquitoes. During the 1950s, nationalist independence movements gained traction across Africa. The movements advanced under various banners and slogans. Some championed the ideology of Marxist liberation and withdrawal from markets controlled by their colonial rulers; others sought democratic rule by the majority and the virtues of the free market; and yet others embraced hazy philosophical programs of "African socialism." In southern and eastern Africa, the movements focused on the immediate goal of forcing out colonial rulers and reclaiming for African populations lands that had been seized by European settlers. During the course of these struggles for independence, many facets of the colonial programs – even those of medical services – came to be disparaged.

Colonial rule ended first in the Gold Coast (now Ghana) in 1957 and then across much of British, French, and Belgian Africa in the early 1960s. Some of the political transitions from European to African rule were accomplished without major disruption; others were chaotic and only achieved through violence. The newly empowered "nationalist" movements were generally organized on the basis of a single political party that, at least in principle, would look after the interests of the peoples who resided within the new states. The African consensus, formulated by the political elites of one-party states, was that other issues would have to take priority over the programs of malaria control that had been inherited from their former colonial rulers.

In the British colony of Southern Rhodesia (now Zimbabwe), European settlers were able to thwart the African independence movement for fifteen years by a unilateral declaration of independence in 1965. After the unilateral declaration, the new Rhodesian regime continued its program of malaria control with limited financial resources, concentrating on the prevention of epidemics. The gains from these programs were partly undone during the last stages of the liberation war, and the summer of 1979–1980 marked the worst malaria season since 1955.[1] The governments of the major Portuguese settler colonies of Angola and Mozambique engaged in counter-insurgency warfare against African independence fighters until the collapse of the military junta in Portugal in 1974; the colonial regimes ceased to exist the following year. In the interim, from 1960 into the early 1970s, the colonial government of Mozambique committed to a World Health Organization (WHO)-sponsored program of pre-eradication malaria control, but these efforts encountered the same problems that had dogged malaria eradication projects in tropical Africa.[2] Beyond these last European colonial regimes, however, there was scant support for the expense and tedium of malaria control. In the surge of enthusiasm for African rule and a new dispensation of natural resources and government largesse, African populations had other priorities.

Economic growth was foremost. Many newly formed African governments committed themselves to increasing economic growth to improve the lives of their African populations. Could it be argued that ongoing malaria control was critically important for African economic growth? Indirect support for this view came from economists who examined the economic evidence from Ceylon (now Sri Lanka). The evidence was mixed. Ceylon had a profoundly different malarial environment than did tropical Africa. Most infections were vivax, and Ceylon had a highland region in which malaria was highly unstable. The Ceylonese populations had suffered a horrific epidemic of malaria in 1935 that had swept away more than 100,000 people, and thus the establishment of malaria control (and near eradication) was at least as significant for adults as for children. In

---

[1] P. Taylor and S. L. Mutambu, "A Review of the Malaria Situation in Zimbabwe with Special Reference to the Period 1972–1981," *Transactions of the Royal Society of Tropical Medicine and Hygiene*, vol. 80, no. 1 (1986), 12–19.

[2] João Fernando Lima Schwalbach and Maria Cecilia Reyes Dela Maza, *A Malária em Moçambique [1937–1973]* (n.p.: Instituto Nacional de Saude, n.d. [circa 1974]), 37–75.

An effort in the mid-1950s to eradicate malaria in the Limpopo valley, a rural region with a population of nonimmune Europeans, had established effective malaria control but was unable to achieve eradication. See Alberto Soeiro, "A Malária em Moçambique, Com Espeical Referência à Campanha Antimalárica Numa Região Predominantemente Urbana (Lourenço Marques) e Uma Região Predominantemente Rural (Vale do Limpopo)," *Anais do Instituto de Medicina Tropical*, vol. 13, no. 4 (1956), 615–634.

Ceylon, the global Malaria Eradication Program had racked up truly impressive reductions in malarial infections. It had lowered death rates and raised childhood survival rates. As a consequence, there were now more mouths to feed per laboring member of the population. On the other hand, economists thought that this impact would be more than outweighed by the reduction in mortality and morbidity among the laboring population. At least over the short term, the net impact was judged to be positive.[3] The implications for tropical Africa were far from clear.

By the mid-1960s, the highly charged expressions of professional judgment over the value of IRS and the potential impact of the loss of immunity, showcased at Kampala in 1950, were long forgotten. The malaria eradication pilot projects had been put to rest. The powerful antimalarial chloroquine was becoming increasingly available in rural Africa. The slate had been wiped clean. The working assumptions of the malaria program officers were that, in the aftermath of unsuccessful projects, once "protected" populations were left no worse off than before the interventions. The status quo ante had simply been re-established. These assumptions fitted comfortably into a broader meta-paradigm of equilibrium analysis that held the day in a number of disciplines, including economics and the emerging field of ecology. From this perspective, the malaria interventions were ephemeral and had no lasting effect on the immunities of human beings or anopheline vectors. It followed without saying that there could be no pressing ethical or medical issues to be investigated.

The economic logic for malaria intervention in the mid to late 1960s was a restatement of that from the 1950s. It stressed the benefits that would accrue to Africans as a consequence of subduing the specter of malaria. It expressed a tendency among public health analysts and economists to extend the lessons of Ceylon to the wider world. Yet, no one undertook an analysis of the African data; thus, the reality that the most critical dimensions of African malarial infections were of childhood mortality

---

[3] Robin Barlow, "The Economic Effects of Malaria Eradication," *American Economic Review*, vol. 57, no. 2 (1967), 130–148. Barlow based his model on data published by Peter Newman in his book *Malaria Eradication and Population Growth with Special Reference to Ceylon and British Guiana* (Ann Arbor: University of Michigan Press, 1965). See also Peter Newman's comments in George H. Borts, Herbert E. Klarman, and Peter Newman, "Discussion," *American Economic Review*, vol. 57, no. 2 (1967), 155–157.
On the history of assessments of the economic impact of malaria, see Randall M. Packard, "'Roll Back Malaria, Roll in Development?': Reassessing the Economic Burden of Malaria," *Population and Development Review*, vol. 35, no. 1 (2009), 53–87.

and childhood morbidities with medical sequelae and disabilities never entered into the equations.

A different line of argument, perhaps implicit in the African interests in other priorities, was that a strong case could be made for investments in economic growth without malaria control. It, too, was made with reference to experiences outside of tropical Africa. Many specialists attributed the decline of malaria in Europe and North America to rising incomes that allowed for better housing and increased access to antimalarial medicines. Might the same not be true for Africans?

At all events, development specialists who gambled on development theory and international bankers who bellied up to the table talked many African leaders into borrowing massive sums and betting their monies on industrial economic growth. In retrospect, it is well recognized that the vast majority of these early investments in industrial growth came to naught. The much-vaunted takeoff into sustained economic growth crashed on the runway. This development disaster had a series of unimagined consequences, among them a crushing debt burden that hampered investments in nonindustrial sectors, including public health. The upside, if there was one, was that the development debacle unfolded during a period in which the export agricultural sector turned in a positive performance. The good years began in the late 1940s and, aided by a positive movement in barter terms of trade during the 1960s, continued into the early 1970s. This made the poor investment policy choices of most African governments – that included massive loans with heavy debt service obligations – less immediately consequential than they would have been otherwise.[4] During the 1960s and early 1970s, African incomes, as measured by macroeconomic indicators such as gross domestic product (GDP) per capita, rose at a modest rate of between 1 and 2 percent per year.[5]

African governments borrowed heavily and focused their investments principally in urban areas, constructing prestigious buildings and state-owned industrial projects, improving their armed forces, and enlarging their state bureaucracies. This had the effect of making urban constituencies

[4] David K. Fieldhouse, *Black Africa, 1945–1980: Economic Decolonization and Arrested Development* (London: Unwin Hyman, 1986), especially 231–246.
[5] Benno J. Ndulu and Stephen A. O'Connell, "Policy Plus: African Growth Performance, 1960–2000," in Benno J. Ndulu, Stephen A. O'Connell, Robert H. Bates, Paul Collier, and Chukwuma C. Soludo (eds.), *The Political Economy of Economic Growth in Africa, 1960–2000*, vol. 1 (New York: Cambridge University Press, 2008), figure 1.3 Smoothed Average Growth in Real GDP Per Capita, 1960–2000 (Countries with a Full Set of Growth Observations), 19.

even more crucial for the survival of these regimes, thus generating a self-reinforcing cycle of investment. This was a critical dynamic in the emergence of the different worlds of urban and rural Africa. As African governments began to focus their expenditures on urban constituencies, they spent their health monies principally on urban, hospital-based, curative services that reached about 15 percent of their populations.[6] And in urban Africa, malaria was far less of a public health problem than in rural Africa, in large measure because there were fewer potential breeding sites for the anopheline mosquitoes. Malaria control in the early decades of the postcolonial period was focused in urban areas, as it had been in the colonial period.

African states did not embrace a commitment to the proposed WHO malaria pre-eradication program, and no master plan for African public health even came under consideration. Some African states – notably, Tanzania – began to build on the rudimentary structure of rural health services developed during the colonial period. Other states took on a hodgepodge of health interventions, largely driven by monies that were made available from international donors to target specific diseases.

Rural populations largely went without mosquito control from the state. There was little if any rural environmental engineering to reduce mosquito habitat, larviciding to reduce mosquito populations, or spraying to reduce adult mosquito populations. In the extensive areas in which effective control had been achieved during the era of the WHO projects, malaria transmission – after the chaotic epidemic rebound – was re-established.

Early in the independence era, African populations continued to have recourse to a wide array of plant-based medicines, some of which had the ability to reduce parasite loads or alleviate some malaria symptoms. These medicines did not clear infections, yet many were palliative. Those with fever-reducing or antiparasitic properties did produce an improvement in health. The therapeutic practices and the medicinal plants that were the basis of the pharmacopoeia of African peoples were highly diverse, and these systems were far from static.[7] When people traveled to find work on a seasonal or permanent basis, moved from village to town or city, or served

---

[6] Meredeth Turshen, *Privatizing Health Services in Africa* (New Brunswick: Rutgers University Press, 1999), 15.

[7] For a comparison of sub-Saharan African and Native American malarial therapeutic practices, see James L. A. Webb, Jr., "On Biomedicine, Transfers of Knowledge, and Malaria Treatments in Eastern North America and Tropical Africa," 53–68.

in the imperial militaries (as had many during the Second World War), they encountered different therapeutic systems. Africans learned, borrowed, and innovated.

Until the 1960s, Africans had limited access to the most efficacious antimalarial drugs. During the colonial era, the colonial authorities had deemed the cinchona alkaloids (including quinine) too limited in supply and too expensive to provide to large numbers of Africans. Programs to grow cinchona trees on African soils and to use a mix of cinchona alkaloids to treat Africans had come to little because the development of synthetic drugs during the war seemed to render the plantations uneconomic, and the antimalaria program of the immediate postwar years had focused on eradication rather than treatment. During the aborted eradication campaign, pyrimethamine – until parasite resistance had compromised its effectiveness – and chloroquine had achieved good therapeutic success. The major problem for Africans was access. Most rural Africans could not get the new drugs unless they lived within the orbit of a mission hospital or clinic or a European-run farm, plantation, or mining operation.

THE MIRACLE OF CHLOROQUINE

Rural access to highly efficacious antimalarial drugs began to improve rapidly during the 1960s. African states and private merchants began to import the astonishingly inexpensive and highly effective antimalarial drug chloroquine, and the drug began to make its way into African markets even in remote rural areas. Indeed, chloroquine was so inexpensive that it did not attract the interest of drug counterfeiters. It became available for purchase in tens of thousands of small shops that offered, among a plethora of other goods, inexpensive basic commodities such as soap, matches, and cooking oil. This improved access was not the result of a new rural health delivery system or any intervention by malaria experts.

There has never been a study of the African (or global) market for chloroquine. As a consequence, we know little about the sources of supply and virtually nothing about the volume of the drug that was imported.[8] This lack of knowledge is a result of many factors. The specialized field of

---

[8] Early in the chloroquine era, the principal source of supply was Switzerland, but apparently the low profit margins encouraged the Swiss to leave the business, and, by the 1960s, Czechoslovakia became a major global supplier. It in turn was replaced by China.

My understanding of this progression is based on an interview in 2008 with Dr. Alan Shapira, who has spent much of his career dealing with malaria.

malariology was in decline by the late 1960s, as the global malaria program failed to achieve the eradication of what was perceived to be the single heaviest disease burden in the world. Mixed success was deemed failure. In the campaign years (1955–1969), when the elixir of potent insecticides promised a universal solution to malarial infection, field entomologists and malaria specialists had been deemed largely superfluous and few trained to take their place. The newly independent African governments concentrated their modest efforts on the improvement of population health in urban areas. The former colonial powers concentrated on securing their economic interests in the newly independent states. There was no large-scale collection of African rural health data. As a result, there was little awareness that African populations had embarked on the single most epidemiologically significant intervention in the history of African malaria to date.

In Senegal, beginning in 1963, the newly independent state distributed chloroquine at a very low price per tablet through the government system of rural cooperatives. The goal was to reach the population up to 14 years of age during the malaria transmission season (extending from July to December) to provide an effective chemoprophylaxis for those who had not acquired effective immunological protection. Most of the chloroquine went for its intended purpose, and the rural population soon embraced its use. Chloroquine consumption in Senegal doubled from 1963 through 1966, to more than 13 million tablets. The health results were spectacular: the number of villagers with measurable parasites or distended spleens declined precipitously, and there was a marked decline in sickness and death owing to malaria. The WHO determined that malaria in Senegal was no longer hyperendemic. At worst, it was mesoendemic, and in the pilot project area where IRS had been used, it was considered hypoendemic. Indeed, the initiative was so successful – and chloroquine was so accessible – that rural populations adopted a new practice of taking chloroquine at the least suspicion of fever, particularly during the transmission season. By the end of the 1966 season, it was estimated that the population would have used 40 million tablets of chloroquine had it been available.[9]

Chloroquine use spread throughout tropical Africa. The details are scant because no one was keeping records of who took what medicine when and in what dosages. But in the aftermath of efforts to control malaria at Pare-Taveta in Tanzania, twenty years after the end of IRS, a

[9] I. Wone and R. Michel, "Bilan de la chemioprophylaxie systématique par chloroquine au Sénégal, 1963–1966," *Médecine d'Afrique Noire*, no. 6, June 1967, 267–269.

malariometric survey revealed that there had been no decline in the density of vectors or in their rates of infectivity. What had markedly declined, however, was morbidity and mortality among the African populations. The authors of the study determined that some of the decline might be attributed to the gradual improvement in health services, particularly for maternal and child health, and some might plausibly be assigned to the use of pyrethrum sprays and mosquito coils. They concluded, however, that the ready availability and use of chloroquine was the most significant factor in the decline in malaria.[10]

The African appreciation of modern antimalarial therapy blended with older beliefs about the disease. In Senegal, where one of the first rural opinion surveys about malaria was conducted in 1966, roughly half of the rural inhabitants surveyed did not know that mosquitoes carried the infection. Those who invoked their folk knowledge of the transmission of the disease variously linked it to the rains, the sun, fog, swamps, or mangoes (that ripen during the transmission season) among other causes. Nearly half of the Senegalese surveyed were keen to take chloroquine and generally were appreciative of the IRS campaigns, as long as the village chiefs had given their authorization. The villagers were not keen, however, to participate in the health propaganda mass meetings that malaria control specialists favored or to provide blood samples to malariologists. They credited those who demanded the frequent blood sampling with ulterior motives.[11]

Chloroquine had a major impact on African health. It seems to have reduced infant and early childhood deaths from malaria by roughly 25–35 percent.[12] This was tremendous solace to families whose children thereby survived the early rounds of parasite infections. Fewer infants and children were buried, and families grew larger. Through their children, African adults secured support for themselves in their later years. In this sense, the bounty of surviving children seemed a pure blessing.

The increase in child survival also had a larger demographic significance. It became one of the important factors in the transformation of the

[10] Y. G. Matola and S. A. Magayuka, "Malaria in the Pare Area of Tanzania. V. Malaria 20 Years after the End of Residual Insecticide Spraying," *Transactions of the Royal Society of Tropical Medicine and Hygiene*, vol. 75, no. 6 (1981), 811–813.

[11] M. Sankale, B. Diop, and I. Gueye, "Enquête d'opinion sur le paludisme en milieu rural au Sénégal," *Médecine d'Afrique Noire*, no. 6, June 1967, 271–280.

[12] There may have been other forces that produced this improvement in survival. The issue is understudied. National childhood vaccination programs in tropical Africa were relatively insignificant before 1980.

age structures of African populations. More infants and young children survived to later childhood and early adulthood than ever before in the history of the African continent. There were now more mouths to feed per adult. This was a drag on economic growth because an increasing percentage of the population was now below the age of productive work. Because virtually all adults had some functional immunity to malaria, the increase in chloroquine use does not appear to have resulted in a major reduction in adult morbidity that would have been expressed in greater economic productivity.

During the 1960s, these profound changes to the age pyramid were occurring during a period of healthy economic growth, and it was possible to be optimistic. Perhaps increased child survival in a period of economic growth would mark the beginning of a "demographic transition," as had taken place in industrialized economies when families realized that they did not require as many children. Perhaps in a primarily agricultural economy, such a demographic transition would be driven by a transformation in ways of life – such as the broader adoption of animal traction or the mechanization of agriculture – that would reduce the need for labor in the fields. Some economic development projects aimed at such goals, but success was elusive.

By the mid-1970s, the WHO estimated that infant and early childhood deaths attributable to malaria had been reduced to 600,000. Chloroquine had played a central role. Effective malaria control using vector control methods could only be achieved in urban areas, mining centers, and on some export-oriented plantations and was principally a continuation of colonial-era programs. Only 17 percent of the population of tropical Africa that was at risk of malaria was thus "protected."[13]

The prospects for a demographic transition gradually dimmed. Beginning in the middle of the decade, across sub-Saharan Africa, the rate of GDP growth began to decline and then turned negative from 1979 to 1995.[14] Several factors influenced this downward spiral. Many

---

[13] USAID, Office of Health, "Report of Consultants–African Malaria [1975]," 2. PN-AAN-885. Available online: http://pdf.usaid.gov/pdf_docs/PNAAN885.pdf. The broadening age pyramid went unnoticed in some sectors of the malaria control community. Some reports, for example, argued without data that African malarial infections and deaths had increased since the waning of the WHO efforts; this made logical sense only if chloroquine access was left out of the picture. See, for example, USAID, Mission to Zaire, "Draft. Review of Malaria Control Programs in Developing Countries: Zaire, Africa Country Summary," 4. PD-ABA-487. November 1981. Available online: http://pdf.usaid.gov/pdf_docs/PDABA487.pdf

[14] Benno J. Ndulu and Stephen A. O'Connell, "Policy Plus," 19.

well-educated Africans left the continent to seek better opportunities abroad. Many African governments undertook new, ill-advised policies of industrialization on the advice of development economists, and many African governments continued to expend most of their scarce resources in the urban sector. To help finance these initiatives, some regimes stripped resources from their agricultural export sectors through the pricing mechanisms of marketing boards that acted as the sole buyers of agricultural products for export. All African governments suffered from a paucity of well-educated bureaucrats, and many government workers succumbed to pressures to give privileges to family members, to supplicants with influence, or to those who offered bribes. The international economic environment was also negatively charged. The net barter terms of trade for many African agricultural goods turned against African producers, and the obligations to service the debt burden that had been incurred during the 1960s and early 1970s were an additional drag on economic performance. The broadening base of the age pyramid deepened the economic crisis, although it was not one of its prime causes. Rural incomes fell. There were more young mouths to feed than ever before.

There were other important public health consequences of chloroquine use beyond child survival. The health of older children and adults improved. Although virtually all older children and adults were protected by some degree of acquired immunity, the use of chloroquine reduced the severity of bouts of malarial fever, boosted attendance at school, and improved the vigor of those in the fields or at other places of work. These were positive advances, set the midst of shifting economic trends.

PRIMARY HEALTH CARE

The political agendas of the new African states that achieved independence in the 1960s did not stress health care. Many of the new states inherited rudimentary public health systems. Malawi, for example, had eighty-four physicians, three dentists, five pharmacists, twenty registered nurses, and one nurse-midwife to serve a population of 3.8 million.[15] Some states were better off than Malawi, and a few – such as Nigeria, Kenya, and Ghana – had schools for training nurses and other health care providers. But even these states had grossly inadequate staff and budgets to provide health services to their newly independent citizens and what resources were

---

[15] Turshen, *Privatizing Health Care in Africa*, 30.

made available to the health services were largely disbursed in urban populations. The mission hospitals and clinics, thin as they were on the ground, continued to play a significant role in treating the rural sick.[16]

The older, colonial model of concentration on the great endemic diseases still held the day into the 1960s, even as malaria eradication projects were shown to be unworkable in tropical Africa. In the wake of the failure of the global malaria eradication program (1955–1969) to realize fully its goal of ridding the globe of the plasmodia that caused human malaria, public health specialists concerned with the burden of disease in the developing world became disenchanted with the idea of targeting a single disease for eradication.[17] Wouldn't far greater improvements in health be achieved through the provision of basic health services to rural populations around the world? Representatives of newly independent states had changed the balance of political power in the World Health Assembly, and, in meetings among public health practitioners and in the offices of policy-making bureaucrats during the mid-1970s, a movement to endorse primary health care (PHC) began to gain traction. It was pushed forward by the Soviet Union, which sought to highlight its own health system. In 1978, at the First International Conference on Primary Health Care, held at Alma Ata, the WHO announced its endorsement of a new model for global health.[18]

The commitment to PHC in many African quarters existed mostly on paper. Any diversification of the African government health systems would depend on a reallocation of resources from cities and towns to the rural sector or an increase in health spending. The primacy of urban politics continued to trump rural health, and there was little if any significant increase in health spending. The prospects for PHC were made even more difficult by the broader downturn in African economic conditions,

---

[16] On the early history of mission hospitals and clinics, see Ralph Schram, *The History of the Nigerian Health Services* (Ibadan: Ibadan University Press, 1971), 59–180. Schram's work covers a much broader field of historical study than his book title indicates.

[17] There was considerable resistance at the highest levels of the WHO to the idea of eradicating smallpox. See D. A. Henderson, *Smallpox: The Death of a Disease* (Amherst, NY: Prometheus Books, 2009), 57–78.

[18] Socrates Litsios, "The Long and Difficult Road to Alma-Ata: A Personal Reflection," *International Journal of Health Services*, vol. 32 (2002), 709–732. A delegation from the United States attended the Alma Ata conference, and the United States endorsed the PHC recommendations along with the other member nations. But state-sponsored PHC for all ran counter to the US market model, in which health care was a commodity to be purchased rather than a right to be extended by the state. Powerful commercial interests in the United States had little interest in accelerating a movement toward universal health care, and the United States came to act as a powerful counterweight to the PHC movement.

including falling per capita incomes and a deterioration in net barter terms of trade.

The ideological shift from the so-called vertical programs that focused on individual diseases to the horizontal system represented by PHC was yet another nail in the coffin of malaria control. Advocates for PHC held that somehow or another malaria control – perhaps through greater access to antimalarial drugs – was compatible with the PHC model. This ran counter to the broad, global experience with malaria control that had refined the templates of how to establish and deploy a malaria control service in which success depended upon specialized and highly trained staff – quite the opposite of the PHC model, which depended upon a cadre of broadly trained health care providers. The very idea of incorporating malaria control into PHC drove malariologists toward despair.[19]

URBANIZATION

As the arc of malaria interventions turned full circle – away from attempts at rural eradication and back to a concentration on urban and high-value economic centers – broad demographic changes reinforced the primacy of cities. Sub-Saharan Africa had an ancient tradition of urbanization. Cities and towns had grown during the precolonial centuries, stimulated by international trade across the Sahara and the Atlantic and Indian Oceans. The colonial period had seen the rise of new port cities and regional markets and a substantial increase in urban populations. Tropical Africa's experience was broadly commensurate with those of other world regions drawn into a thickening web of commercial exchanges, although its integration had lagged that of most world regions by several centuries. Africa during the first wave of political independence remained the most rural of all major world regions.

From the 1960s forward, however, the process of urbanization accelerated. More rural Africans began to migrate to urban centers. The percentage of the total population in tropical Africa living in urban areas increased dramatically – more than doubling – between 1950 and 1980. Powered by in-migration and the demographic surge of the second half of the twentieth century, the number of African urban dwellers increased by more than 400 percent. Tropical Africa became the most

---

[19] USAID, Office of Health, "Report of Consultants–African Malaria [1975]," 16. PN-AAN-885. Available online: http://pdf.usaid.gov/pdf_docs/PNAAN885.pdf

TABLE 4.1. *Urban Populations by Region in Tropical Africa, 1950–1980*

	Total Urban Population		Percentage of Total Population in Urban Areas	
	1950	1980	1950	1980
Eastern Africa	3,405,000	21,605,000	5	15
Central Africa	3,747,000	16,098,000	14	31
Western Africa	6,457,000	36,387,000	10	26

Source: "Table 5.3. Urban Population Estimates and Projections of Africa, by Region, 1950–2025," in H. Max Miller and Ram N. Singh, "Urbanization during the Postcolonial Days," in James D. Tarver (ed.), *Urbanization in Africa: A Handbook* (Westport, Conn.: Greenwood Press, 1994), 69.

rapidly urbanizing region in the world in the second half of the twentieth century.[20] See Table 4.1.

The overall health impacts of African urbanization were surprising and salubrious. Based on fifty-nine health and demographic surveys conducted from 1988 to 2002, researchers discovered that African urban populations enjoyed better general health status than those in rural settings. Infant mortality and childhood mortality rates, for example, were lower in urban than in rural populations.[21]

[20] These impressive demographic forces, however, did not create the largest regional percentage of total population living in urban areas owing to the initially low levels of urbanization in tropical Africa.

The large-scale movement of rural Africans to cities and towns was only one of the major population movements. There was also considerable rural–rural, urban–urban, and urban–rural migration. See Polly Hill, *Development Economics on Trial: The Anthropological Case for a Prosecution* (Cambridge, 1986).

These migrations undoubtedly brought about a heightened degree of inter-regional mixing of the different genotypes of parasite infections that had begun in an earlier era through the displacement of captives during the slave trade era. The details are unrecoverable, but it seems likely that any subregional specificity of falciparum genotypes was blurred in the comings and goings of waves of African labor migrants. To cite only one example: hundreds of thousands of workers from Mali and Upper Volta (now Burkina Faso) flowed each year into the peanut basin of Senegal and the Gambia and returned home at the end of the agricultural season. They brought infections from the peanut fields back to their sending villages and brought their village infections with them when they next departed for seasonal work. Other intraregional patterns of urban–urban, urban–rural, and rural–urban population movements accomplished much the same result. On the seasonal migrations to Senegal and the Gambia, see Philippe David, *Les navétanes: Histoire des migrants saisonniers de l'arachide en Sénégambie des origines à nos jours* (Dakar: Nouvelles Éditions Africaines, 1980).

[21] Hay, S. I., C. A. Guerra, A. J. Tatem, P. M. Atkinson, and R. W. Snow, "Tropical Infectious Diseases: Urbanization, Malaria Transmission, and the Disease Burden in Africa," *Nature Reviews Microbiology*, vol. 3 (January 2005), 82–83. The authors write that the surveys

This urban–rural health differential was in high profile with regard to malaria. Urban dwellers received far fewer infective bites than those who lived in rural areas.[22] In good measure, this was because anopheline mosquitoes in Africa found it difficult to breed in towns and cities.[23] The anophelines needed clean freshwater breeding habitat, and these habitats were in short supply. The growth of urban settlements sharply reduced the prospects for freshwater breeding through the conversion of habitat to other uses and through the pollution of what breeding sites remained.[24] This process of habitat loss dramatically reduced the densities of vector mosquitoes. And because urban areas were densely settled, the overall result was a steep decline in malaria exposure per capita.[25] In the late 1960s, in Bathurst (now Banjul), the capital of Republic of the Gambia, an assessment of endemic malaria in children indicated a very low rate of parasitemia of 2.5 percent, in comparison to a rate of 76 percent in Jali, an interior village. There was little IRS practiced in Bathurst; the principal antimosquito measure was a fortnightly spraying of insecticide with a fogging machine.[26]

The loss of mosquito breeding habitat and an increase in pollution contributed to an improvement in human health in terms of malaria morbidity

"show that, compared with those living in rural areas, mothers and children living in urban communities have better nutritional status indicators; fewer morbid events; increased vaccine coverage; better physical access to health services; and greater use of insecticide-treated nets (ITN)."

[22] The generalized understandings masked some significant differentials between poor urban inhabitants with inadequate living conditions in high transmission zones and poor urban inhabitants with inadequate living conditions living in low transmission zones, as well as the roughly 60 percent of all urban residents who had adequate living conditions, regardless of the level of transmission in the surrounding or peri-urban areas. J. Keiser, J. Utzinger, M. Caldas de Castro, T.A. Smith, M. Tanner, and B.H. Singer, "Urbanization in Sub-Saharan Africa and Implication for Malaria Control," *American Journal of Tropical Medicine and Hygiene*, vol. 71, supplement 2 (2004), 118–127.

[23] In recent years, anophelines have begun to adapt to some polluted urban environments. In Bobo-Dioulasso, *Anopheles arabiensis* has adapted to highly polluted sites. See Christopher M. Jones, Hyacinthe K. Toé, Antoine Sanou, Moussa Namountougou, Angela Hughes, Abdoulaye Diabaté, Roch Dabiré, Frederic Simard, and Hilary Ranson, "Additional Selection for Insecticide Resistance in Urban Malaria Vectors: DDT Resistance in *Anopheles arabiensis* from Bobo-Dioulasso, Burkina Faso," *PLOS ONE*, vol. 9, no. 9 (2012), 1–9.

[24] A consequence of the loss of anopheline habitat in Tanzania was an increase of nuisance mosquitoes, such as *Culex pipens fatigans*, that breed in polluted waters. (Y.H. Bang, F.M. Mrope, and I.B. Sabuni, "Changes in Mosquito Populations Associated with Urbanization in East Africa," *East African Medical Journal*, vol. 54, no. 7 (1977), 403–410.)

[25] Hay et al., "Tropical Infectious Diseases," 83–84.

[26] G. Harverson and M.E. Wilson, "Assessment of Current Malarial Endemicity in Bathurst, Gambia," *West African Medical Journal*, vol. 17 (1968), 63–67.

and mortality. The sharp decline in the number of infective bites per annum translated into fewer malarial crises, fewer deaths, and less debility. This positive outcome was principally a result of the ecologies of unplanned settlement, rather than of programs of malarial intervention. In some areas, local governments did undertake the routine larviciding of anopheline breeding sites, but the effectiveness of such efforts depended on extensive monitoring and oversight, and this was often lacking. Routine larviciding was carried forward, for example, in Kaduna, Nigeria, yet visiting malariologists who assessed these efforts on behalf of US Agency for International Development (USAID) concluded that the control measures had a negligible impact on the mosquito problem.[27]

A SEARCH FOR OPTIONS

During the late 1960s and 1970s, malaria in Africa was largely uncontrolled by national or international health interventions. Few countries had committed funds to malaria control. Nigeria was the outstanding leader in this regard, with US$30 million allocated for malaria in 1975, although without a plan for how to use these funds.[28] In independent Tanzania, the anopheline control program of the former British colony, deployed in fifty-seven settlements, fell into decline.[29]

At some small, economically important sites such as mining communities, a mix of malaria control strategies succeeded in keeping the rates of infection low. In the town of Yekepa, Liberia, the mining company LAMCO Joint Venture launched a malaria control program in 1963. It included IRS (from 1965 to 1969, when it was abandoned owing to its cost and then recommenced in 1976), environmental engineering (draining and filling of mosquito habitat), and chemoprophylaxis. A company hospital provided free medical care for employees and allowed for rapid diagnosis and treatment. The spleen rate of African children in Yekepa was 10.7 percent; that of children in the surrounding area was 95 percent. Malaria control produced an island of hypoendemicity in a sea of holoendemic infection.[30]

[27] USAID, Office of Health, "Report of Consultants–African Malaria [1975]," 12. PN-AAN-885. Available online: http://pdf.usaid.gov/pdf_docs/PNAAN885.pdf
[28] USAID, Office of Health, "Report of Consultants–African Malaria [1975]," 11. PN-AAN-885. Available online: http://pdf.usaid.gov/pdf_docs/PNAAN885.pdf
[29] Bang, Mrope, and Sabuni, "Changes in Mosquito Populations," 404.
[30] P. Hedman, J. Brohult, J. Forslund, V. Sirleaf, and E. Bengtsson, "A Pocket of Controlled Malaria in a Holoendemic Region of West Africa," *Annals of Tropical Medicine and Parasitology*, vol. 73, no. 4 (1979), 317–325.

At the WHO, the malariologists' hope was to try again to develop protocols that would succeed in malaria eradication – using the same tools that had achieved impressive, if ephemeral, success during the era of the pilot projects. From the mid-1960s into the mid-1970s, just before the success of the PHC movement, the WHO undertook a number of experimental projects in West Africa to refine the approaches to using IRS, sometimes in combination with mass drug administration. These programs employed the same basic approaches as had the pilot projects, and they achieved the same basic results.

In the savanna region of Anécho district, Togo, a malaria control demonstration project employed two annual rounds of IRS to cover a population of 207,000. The project began in 1965. Great improvements in the parasitological indices were noted until the emergence of DDT resistance in 1968. In Kankiya, in northern Nigeria, DDT spraying was combined with mass drug administration. During the two years of the project, it proved possible to achieve a substantial degree of control, but it was again found to be impossible to interrupt transmission. In the forest zone, in Palimé district, Togo, in both dense and degraded forests, an annual spraying of DDT produced vector resistance within three months. Near Kisumu, Kenya, a new insecticide, fenitrothion, was deployed without success. In the judgment of the WHO entomologist A. R. Zahar, "residual house spraying cannot be considered as a principal tool for long-term malaria control in tropical Africa." Short of eradication, the answer seemed to be a mix of strategies that included chemical therapy; source reduction; biological controls, such as antilarval fish and antimosquito bacteria; and personal protection through the use of bed nets, screens, and antimosquito coils; in addition, programs had to be tailored to the local environments.[31]

THE GARKI PROJECT

In the late 1960s, the WHO initiated its last malaria eradication pilot project in sub-Saharan Africa. Many of the earlier pilot projects had been poorly documented, and some malariologists interpreted the summary project reports to mean that the technical, administrative, financial, and epidemiological problems encountered in these early projects were

[31] A. R. Zahar, "Vector Control Operations in the African Context," *Bulletin of the World Health Organization*, vol. 62, supplement (1984), 89–100. Quotation from page 92.

surmountable – at least in the more humid zones, in which transmission was stable.[32] It was abundantly clear, however, that projects undertaken in the savanna and sahelian regions had not achieved the full interruption of transmission. Were the earlier projects' shortcomings remediable? Would it be possible to mount a new offensive against *Plasmodium falciparum* in the sahel, document the project thoroughly, identify shortcomings, and press an attack until full interruption of transmission was achieved?

The WHO identified a site in northern Nigeria and, in 1969, in league with the Nigerian government, began to plan a full-out attack on malaria. It was more thoroughly prosecuted than any earlier pilot project, yet the overall findings were depressingly familiar. Even with the assiduous application of insecticide in combination with mass drug administration, it was not possible to interrupt the transmission of malaria. The project analysis was elegant, a testament to the high level of professionalism of the project staff, yet there were limitations to the project's findings. The malariologists noticed that there had been a considerable reduction in morbidity and mortality, particularly as a result of mass drug administration, but this could not be quantified. And the malariologists intuited that the short-term steep reduction in malaria transmission had probably not exacted a cost in the loss of clinical immunity for the simple reason that it had only lasted eighteen months.[33]

As in the earlier pilot projects, the hopes for malaria eradication at Garki had been pinned principally on the remarkable efficacy of IRS in combination with mass drug administration. The logic of IRS was built on the assumption that malarial vectors took their human blood meals indoors. The Garki project documented that a subset of anopheline vectors took their blood meals outdoors and were thus not susceptible to IRS.

NO CLEAR PATH AHEAD

International donors grew discouraged. The prospects of relaunching a broad IRS campaign were extremely poor, owing to a lack of African

---

[32] On the early Liberian projects, see James L. A. Webb, Jr., "The First Large-Scale Use," 347–376.

[33] There was, however, a partial loss of parasitological immunity by the end of the eighteen-month intervention. Louis Molineaux and Gabriele Gramiccia, *The Garki Project: Research on the Epidemiology and Control of Malaria in the Sudan Savanna of West Africa* (Geneva: World Health Organization, 1980), 292–294.

interest and to rising insecticide prices. In 1970, the Malaria Program of the US Centers for Disease Control, whose charge was to help developing countries eliminate malaria by providing technical and financial assistance, was active in eighteen countries. Not one was in tropical Africa.[34]

Specialists sought workable solutions but encountered formidable social and political issues that lay outside of their fields of technical training. A proposal to encourage African communities to take on a program of self-help that included screening, bed nets, pyrethrum coils and sprays, and antimalarial drugs would have to negotiate in the grand diversity of African rural societies. What seemed possible in the compact villages of northern Nigeria, in which village chiefs and emirs exercised hierarchical control, seemed impossible in the dispersed individual compounds of Kenya.[35]

In 1976, the United States launched a malaria control program in three of twenty-four urban zones in Kinshasa, Zaire, as well as in a small rural area nearby. It was, in the late 1970s, the only US malaria control program in sub-Saharan Africa. It was declared nonreplicable in 1981. During the short life of the program, some 300,000 urban dwellers and 7,775 rural dwellers were protected by IRS using DDT. The impetus for the project came entirely from the Americans because the government of Zaire had no national health plan and little functioning national health infrastructure. By 1981, the Americans had decided to integrate all future antimalaria measures into the PHC system. There were two problems: the PHC system existed in name only, and the need for specialists to carry out vector control measures was a misfit with the PHC model.[36]

A broader review of the African malarial situation by the American Public Health Association in 1982 reiterated the consensus of malaria control specialists in the decade before the Kampala Conference in 1950:

Vector control which includes wide-spread chemical control will in Africa be appropriate only in localized areas, for protection of urban and periurban

[34] US Department of Health, Education, and Welfare, *Annual Report. Fiscal Year 1970. Malaria Program, Center for Disease Control* (Atlanta: CDC, 1970), iii.
[35] USAID, Office of Health, "Report of Consultants–African Malaria [1975]," 29–31. PN-AAN-885. Available online: http://pdf.usaid.gov/pdf_docs/PNAAN885.pdf
[36] USAID, Mission to Zaire, "Draft. Review of Malaria Control Programs," 15, 29–32.

populations; in some of the coastal islands; or under specialized circumstances such as the need to protect strategic areas or groups for economic, social, or political reasons. In such circumstances, operational responsibility of vector control should wherever possible be decentralized to such administrative units as municipalities or productive enterprises. Such activity as chemical control or large-scale environmental management will usually require planning at a higher level, with technical inputs and support from a specialized vector control unit.[37]

What realistically could be done? In 1979, WHO experts weighed the constraints and developed four "tactical variants" for malaria control. Tactical variant I was deemed the most critical and demanded the fewest resources. It promoted chloroquine use to prevent death in pregnant women and young children, the populations most at risk. The de facto policy was an expansion of access to chloroquine through rural clinics that supplemented the chloroquine available in rural shops. Some experts thought that access to chloroquine might be further expanded to provide mass prophylaxis programs for the under-five age group to reduce mortality.[38]

Malaria deaths were declining as a result of increased access to antimalarial drugs – principally chloroquine – and accelerating urbanization. There was, however, serious trouble ahead. By the late 1970s, resistance to chloroquine was widespread in Southeast Asia. The prospect of the emergence of resistance in tropical Africa boded poorly: if chloroquine were to become ineffective, tactical variant I would stumble into insignificance. There was no back-up drug to chloroquine, and no new drug development was in the pipeline.

DAMS AND IRRIGATION PROJECTS

As African populations grew in absolute numbers and became younger, African agricultural production per capita declined. African states began

---

[37] American Public Health Association, "Workshop Report. Malaria Control in PHC in Africa. Washington, DC, June 28–July 2, 1982," 19. Available online: http://pdf.usaid.gov/pdf_docs/PNAAY965.pdf

[38] The author of a 1984 WHO assessment of African progress on the "plans of action" concluded that the evidence was so fragmentary and incomplete that no critical review was possible. E. G. Beausoleil, "A Review of Present Antimalarial Activities in Africa," *Bulletin of the World Health Organization*, vol. 62, supplement (1984), 14–15.

In the early 1980s, at least eight countries (Benin, Comoros, the Gambia, Mali, Niger, Togo, United Republic of Tanzania, and Upper Volta) received free supplies of chloroquine for two years from the Arab Gulf Programme for United Nations Development Organization [AGFUND]. (Beausoleil, "Review of Present Antimalarial Activities," 14.)

to import food to provision their urban populations, and the food imports were so inexpensive that they undercut the ability of African farmers to compete. Most African farming compounds produced food for their own needs and, when the financial prospects were promising, they grew cash crops for export or sent young workers to seek jobs in the cities or abroad. African urban populations grew much faster than rural populations, and urban populations became increasingly less dependent upon local farmers for their food.

The water resources of Africa were as yet largely undeveloped, and economic planners turned their attention to them. Dams would allow for irrigated agriculture and hydropower. Impounded water could be used to improve the production of food crops. The water could also be used to irrigate cash crops, thus increasing yields and bolstering the economic position of African states.

According to the economic orthodoxy of the 1960s and 1970s, African states were encouraged to try to achieve a balance between food crops and cash crops, to strive for "food self-sufficiency." Economic planners from industrialized countries proposed large development schemes to dramatically increase African food production. In theory, this would improve the economic position of African states by reducing their dependence on food imports. The increase in food production would also, in theory, reduce the vulnerability of African populations to famine.

The large-scale dams and irrigation projects were seductive on paper. Economists calculated positive rates of return on investment, engineers drew up detailed blueprints, and economists and engineers determined that African farmers and migrant laborers would reap large benefits from improved water control. Africans laboring in the irrigation programs would produce food surpluses to feed the cities. Africans living in cities and towns would eat the food and would reap the benefits of inexpensive electricity produced by the dams' turbines and transmitted over long-distance power lines. This would reduce many African states' dependence on imported energy.

Few funders realized that the Africans themselves had gone missing from the plans for African development. What worked in Tennessee was erroneously assumed to be workable in Senegal. The development plans did not include assessments of the costs to villagers forcibly displaced by the filling up of reservoirs and who were thereby impoverished, and this contributed to the planners' overestimation of economic benefits. These blinkered perspectives were part of a larger cultural shift that elevated the mathematically oriented sciences above others. There was also, however, a fundamental linguistic divide. The development planners literally did not speak the languages of those for whom they purportedly planned. In retrospect, the hubris was breathtaking.[39]

It was also dangerous. The planned interventions involved major transformations of local and regional ecologies, and the disease consequences of these interventions were largely ignored.[40] In some regions, the impounded waters created vast habitat for snails, flies, and mosquitoes, even while human populations were settled around the impounded waters to work in the irrigated perimeters. The disease mix varied according to local ecologies. Commonly, the result was an increase in the transmission of schistosomiasis, onchocerciasis, and malaria.

In arid lands, the year-round impoundment of water supplies also transformed the patterns of malaria transmission. Around the Manatali dam in Mali, for example, the starkly seasonal pattern of transmission lengthened to one of year-round transmission.[41] In the vast Gezira-Managil irrigation projects in the Sudan along the Blue Nile, the expansion of irrigation produced a new bimodal distribution of malaria transmission. The previous transmission pattern had occurred during a rainy season that lasted from August or September until December (with a peak in September and October). During the 1960s and 1970s, with an expansion of cotton and wheat production using irrigation, a second peak of malaria transmission occurred in February and March and often carried over until the rainy season began again, in a pattern of (nearly) year-round malaria transmission.[42] In the mid 1970s, a serious malaria epidemic ripped through the Gezira-Managil projects. The large-scale use of pesticides on the agricultural fields had likely selected for resistance in the vector mosquitoes. The epidemic was eventually brought under control through the use of IRS, by which time the mosquitoes were becoming resistant to HCH, DLD, DDT, and malathion.[43]

---

[39] For a broad reflection on this issue, see James C. Scott, *Seeing Like a State: How Certain Schemes to Improve the Human Condition Have Failed* (New Haven, CT: Yale University Press, 1999), 262–306.

[40] William Jobin, *Dams and Disease: Ecological Design and Health Impacts of Large Dams, Canals, and Irrigation Systems* (London: E and FN Spon Press, 1999).

[41] Jobin, *Dams and Disease*, 218–219.

[42] Jobin, *Dams and Disease*, 325.

[43] Jobin, *Dams and Disease*, 335.

EARLY EFFORTS TO DEVELOP A MALARIA VACCINE

The broad disappointments of the global malaria eradication campaign – and the significant impediments to moving ahead even with "pre-eradication" campaigns in Africa that were based on bolstering the capacity for malaria control – led researchers to the view that malaria eradication could not be achieved with the tools at hand. A high level of control in some environments was possible but expensive, and absent the exercise of immediate political power, such control would depend on an African willingness to undertake the work. In the aftermath of political independence for the colonies, the erstwhile imperial powers refashioned their ties with the new African states. Great Britain and France continued to fund their research institutes and centers in the former colonies, and medical research on malaria was ongoing. But there was little interest in continuing to support malaria control. Beset by other pressing concerns, former colonial powers opted for different roles. In the postcolonial era, their influence shrank.

The new powers that might have potentially overshadowed France and Great Britain in Africa were the United States and the Soviet Union, the leaders of two power blocs that squared off against each other in the Cold War. In Africa, the two world powers chose to struggle by proxy, funding leaders who espoused ideologies that were compatible with their own or who would simply accede to their requests. Neither global giant deemed malaria in Africa to be a priority.

Malaria control languished. As the first broad wave of independence washed over the former colonies, the US Congress lost interest in funding the WHO malaria eradication campaign by 1960, and US funds to the WHO malaria account dried up in 1963.[44] Malaria eradication could not be achieved in the tropics, and the US military's experience with malaria in Vietnam convinced military authorities that prophylactic antimalarial drugs could not assure the full protection of nonimmune troops fighting in malarial areas. The damage from malaria could be limited but not fully prevented, and this fed a Cold War fear that US troops might not be combat ready.[45]

---

[44] J. A. Nájera, "Tropical Diseases and Socioeconomic Development," *Parassitologia*, vol. 36 (1994), 17–33.

[45] This fear had deeper roots as well. During the early years of the Second World War, the burden of malaria had been nearly crushing for Allied troops in the Pacific and Asian theaters of war until the adoption of the antimalarial atabrine that replaced the venerable quinine. Even with atabrine, Allied troops had suffered considerable losses to malaria, and a major wartime malaria control program – Malaria Control in War Areas (MCWA) – had

Early in the first eradication era, a malaria vaccine had been generally regarded as an impossible dream: too expensive to develop, unlikely to achieve an improvement over naturally acquired immunity, possibly unsuitable for children in target populations, and likely only useful as an adjunct to IRS and chemical therapy. In 1961, the prospects for a vaccine seemed to improve suddenly. From the U.K. Medical Research Council's Gambian Research Unit came evidence that Gambians infected with malaria produced more gamma globulin than did nonimmune Europeans. Ian McGregor undertook experiments that indicated that people who were infected with malaria produced gamma globulin as part of an immune response that was capable of restricting clinical illness and the density of parasites in their blood. He discovered that their immunity, if only short-lived, could be transferred to nonimmune individuals via their gamma globulin. The floodgates opened.[46]

In 1966, the US government began to fund laboratory research to develop a new tool to solve the malaria problem once and for all. Its success would be measured by how completely it protected nonimmunes from infection. The gold standard was 100 percent protection for US troops in malarial areas. In Washington, the quest for a malaria vaccine came to be conceived of as a matter of national security readiness.

University researchers developed new lines of investigation, and they repeatedly promised breakthroughs that never arrived. USAID developed a Malaria Immunology and Vaccine Research (MIVR) program and lavished millions of dollars annually on the search for a malaria vaccine, ignoring the advice of the broader scientific community in its funding decisions. The USAID MIVR network became tangled up in criminal investigations, charges of sexual harassment, and indictments and convictions for fraud and malfeasance. These problems continued from the mid-1960s into the late 1980s. The USAID MIVR program manipulated and falsified peer review evaluations and expanded its malaria vaccine development projects.[47]

Many promises had been broken. There was no malaria vaccine at hand, and in Africa, childhood survival rates began to slip backward.

---

been undertaken. The Centers for Disease Control (CDC) was a direct outgrowth of the MCWA. On the origins of the CDC, see Justin A. Andrews, "The United States Public Health Service Communicable Disease Center," *Public Health Reports*, vol. 61, no. 33 (1946), 1203–1210.

[46] A comprehensive overview of vaccine development is presented in Irwin W. Sherman, *The Elusive Malaria Vaccine: Miracle or Mirage?* (Washington, DC: ASM Press, 2009). On McGregor in the Gambia, see 111–114.

[47] Sherwin, *The Elusive Malaria Vaccine*, 131–157.

5

Silent Resurgence

The final decades of the twentieth century were marked by dramatic economic, political, and epidemiological change that had direct consequences for malaria control in tropical Africa. The ascension of a new conservative economic orthodoxy in the United States during the presidency of Ronald Reagan shifted policy for health care in most African states toward a "free market" approach. The ongoing struggle against apartheid in Southern Africa and the outbreak of warfare in West and Central Africa made effective malaria control in these regions practically impossible. At the same time, parasite resistance to the front-line antimalarial, chloroquine, began to spread across the continent.

Rural malaria in tropical Africa gathered its forces quietly and resurged almost soundlessly. The continental pandemic hurried large numbers of children to the grave. This resurgence was initially hidden in plain sight. It took place during an era in which death rates for children and adults were in decline, and most experts thought that African societies were in the midst of the "health transition," which was understood to be the first stage in the larger "demographic transition."[1] In retrospect, it is clear that childhood deaths from malaria diverged sharply from the overall trend. Malaria was responsible for approximately 18 percent of all-cause

---

[1] Michel Garenne and Enéas Gakusi, "Health Transitions in Sub-Saharan Africa: Overview of Mortality Trends in Children under 5 Years Old (1950–2000)," *Bulletin of the World Health Organization*, vol. 84, no. 6 (2006), 472; Debbie Bradshaw and Ian M. Timaeus, "Levels and Trends of Adult Mortality," in Dean T. Jamison, Richard G. Feacham, Malegapuru W. Makgoba, Eduard R. Bos, Florence K. Baingana, Karen J. Hofman, and Khama O. Rogo (eds.), *Disease and Mortality in Sub-Saharan Africa* (Washington, DC: World Bank, 2006), 31–42.

childhood mortality in the period before 1960. From 1960 until the end of the 1980s – during the era of chloroquine efficacy, the extension of some basic health care services that included the ready availability of inexpensive oral rehydration therapies, and increased vaccination coverage – malaria deaths declined to 12 percent of all-cause childhood mortality, a decline of one-third in share. But from 1990 to 1995, at the end of the era of chloroquine efficacy, malaria childhood deaths jumped to 30 percent of all-cause mortality.[2]

A LOW PRIORITY

The resurgence took hold during an era in which few African governments monitored malaria and the extension of African health care services to the rural poor was not high on their lists of political priorities. With few exceptions, African governments were principally concerned with the urban constituencies that were a major key to political stability. There was, moreover, little pressure from external forces to address the destruction caused by malaria.

The governments of many tropical African states with "open market" economies continued to pursue economic policies that encouraged the export of agricultural products and minerals to world markets. New and old debt obligations accumulated, and the African governments largely ignored the fiscal problems that metastasized during the slow economic growth of the 1970s and early 1980s. There was little incentive for them to do otherwise. The ongoing political struggle between the socialist and capitalist blocs encouraged Western international aid agencies and international development and financial organizations to extend poorly collateralized loans; to countenance fiscal improprieties, unproductive investments, and human rights abuses; and to continue to provide financial assistance. In the case of Zaire (now the Democratic Republic of Congo), the United States was willing to stand mute during the massive plundering of the country's resources by President Sese Seko Mobutu. It was, at the time, the most spectacular instance of kleptocracy on a continent beleaguered by politicians who exported their ill-gotten personal fortunes.

The quasi-Marxist states – those that found inspiration in communist or socialist policies or that pursued their own paths toward African socialism – were freer to innovate with health policies, and some did. The outstanding

[2] Robert W. Snow, Jean-François Trape, and Kevin Marsh, "The Past, Present, and Future of Childhood Malaria Mortality in Africa," *Trends in Parasitology*, vol. 17, no. 2 (2001), 594.

examples were in southeastern Africa. Tanzania, under the guidance of President Julius Nyerere, extended a rudimentary PHC system into the countryside, reaching millions in rural communities. Mozambique, following its revolutionary struggle against Portuguese colonialism, launched a similar program, but it collapsed under the weight of a civil war funded by South Africa, in which the rebel group RENAMO targeted rural health services for destruction. Zimbabwe, following its independence in 1980, made strong progress in extending health services to rural communities, although these gains were largely reversed during the later years of President Robert Mugabe's increasingly dictatorial rule. (See Map 5.1.)

A NEW ECONOMIC ORTHODOXY

In the United States, Ronald Reagan decisively won the presidential election in 1980 and a new political discourse gained currency. The poor economic performance of the US economy in the late 1970s, rocked as it was by rapid increases in energy prices, was blamed on excessive government interference with the economy. In the United States, it became accepted fact in Republican political circles that the federal government was to blame for unemployment, inflation, and other economic ills. This vision of the dysfunctionality and superfluousness of government was disseminated to the World Bank and International Monetary Fund (IMF), and, in short order, there were calls to reform African governments by shrinking the public sector and promoting private enterprise. The demands became strident and effective when the Soviet Union slid into severe financial and political crisis, and Cold War concerns no longer held pride of place in policy making.

By the mid 1980s, these demands for structural reforms were translated into requirements for African governments to reduce public spending if they were to continue to receive funds from the IMF to forestall bankruptcy. The result was dramatic. In many public sectors, African government jobs and services were reduced. This was not, however, the case in the health sector. In fact, many African governments spent more on health services, although with a decidedly urban focus that targeted patients who were not poor.

In line with a policy advocated by the World Bank, many African governments introduced user fees for health services. The user fees reduced the affordability of health services for the poor, and some of the revenues were used to cover nonsalary items and to maintain facilities for urban

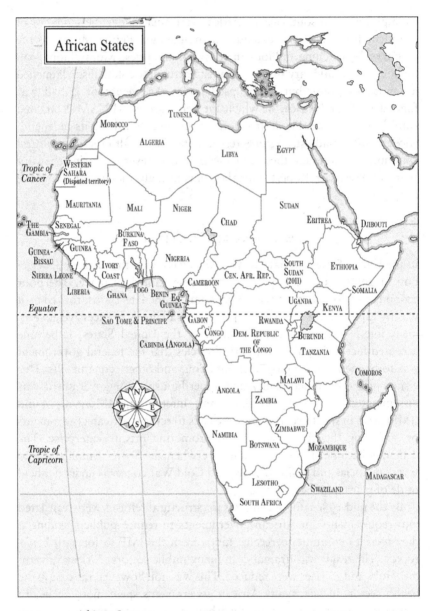

MAP 5.1. African States
Adapted from Roland Oliver, *The African Experience* (New York: HarperCollins, 1991), 233.

populations.[3] The overall picture was that the prior bias toward urban, curative, hospital-based services continued, and the health status of rural African populations deteriorated. The spindly infrastructure of rural clinics came under crushing financial pressure. Some clinics closed and in others key medicines disappeared from the shelves and were not replaced. Even in some urban hospitals, the provision of services was similarly constricted. In Conakry, for example, the hospital staff were paid less than a living wage and had to raise funds from those who needed services. Many in need were turned away because they were desperately poor. Mozambique and Zimbabwe were exceptions, taking significant steps to reorient their budget spending to increase primary and preventive activities.[4]

The World Health Organization (WHO), dependent on contributions from its member states, continued to issue its advisory opinions and maintained its moral authority, although it lost its preeminent position as the arbiter of global health policy. The World Bank took on the challenge. In 1985, it made monies available for investments in the health sectors of developing African nations, with the goal of institutionalizing a market model of health care in tropical Africa. A few African states – Botswana, Nigeria, and Zimbabwe – produced detailed health planning documents. Across most of tropical Africa, the efforts to reorient the allocation of health resources to reach rural populations faced severe economic constraints. Zimbabwe succeeded in effecting a modest reorientation from medical care programs to preventive programs and services. Botswana, bolstered by robust economic growth, succeeded in reaching most of its rural populations. But, in general, African government commitments to the PHC principles of Alma Ata remained largely symbolic.[5] The

---

[3] For studies of the impact of user fees in Ghana, see C. J. Waddington and K. A. Enyimayew, "A Price to Pay: The Impact of User Charges in Ashanti-Akim District, Ghana," *International Journal of Health Planning and Management*, vol. 4 (1989), 17–47; Catriona Waddington and K. A. Enyimayew, "A Price to Pay, Part 2: The Impact of User Charges in the Volta Region of Ghana," *International Journal of Health Planning and Management*, vol. 5 (1990), 287–312.

[4] David Sahn and Rene Bernier, "Have Structural Adjustments Led to Health Sector Reform in Africa?," *Health Policy*, vol. 32, nos. 1–3 (1995), 193–214; Lucy Gilson and Anne Mills, "Health Sector Reforms in Sub-Saharan Africa: Lessons of the Last 10 Years," *Health Policy*, vol. 32, nos. 1–3 (1995), 215–243.

[5] Kwesi Dugbatey, "National Health Policies: Sub-Saharan African Case Studies (1980–1990)," *Social Science & Medicine*, vol. 49, no. 2 (1999), 224–226. Dugbatey chose four states (Botswana, Ivory Coast, Ghana, and Zimbabwe) for his comparative study. Forty of the forty-seven sub-Saharan African states did not have health policy documents with enough substance to allow for analysis.

United Nations Development Report 1991 estimated that more than half of all sub-Saharan Africans had no access to modern medicine.[6]

NEW DIRECTIONS IN MALARIA CONTROL

What were the implications for malaria control? The US Agency for International Development (USAID) commissioned a "Manual on Malaria Control in Primary Health Care in Africa" from the American Public Health Association in 1982; this document adopted the recommendations of the WHO Seventeenth Expert Committee Report (1979).[7] The foundational recommendation, "Tactical Variant I," aimed to reduce mortality through the broader use of chloroquine. The other three variants were more ambitious, combining mortality and morbidity reduction in Tactical Variant II, and moving to progressively more ambitious comprehensive malaria control in Tactical Variants III and IV.[8] In tropical Africa, the best that could be hoped for was Tactical Variant II. This placed the principal emphasis on the chemotherapeutic use of antimalarial drugs at a time when the threat of resistance to these drugs was on the rise. At least in principle, the expansion of PHC networks would provide increased access to antimalarials. The constraints to the successful implementation of such networks, however, were considerable. A low level of economic development and the lack of a clear national health policy, sound health manpower policy, and suitable planning impeded progress in the national and provincial arenas. A raft of other issues shackled the best efforts of the PHC units.[9]

The Americans moved forward from 1982–1993 with a broad new program called the Africa Child Survival Initiative – Combating Childhood Communicable Diseases (CCCD) with the participation of thirteen sub-Saharan African states.[10] It concentrated on reductions in childhood

---

[6] United Nations Development Program, *Human Development Report 1991* (New York: Oxford University Press, 1991), 36.

[7] WHO, Technical Report Series, no. 640. *Seventeenth Report of the WHO Expert Committee on Malaria* (Geneva, 1979).

[8] American Public Health Association, *Manual on Malaria Control in Primary Health Care in Africa* (Washington, DC: Bureau for Africa, USAID, 1982).

[9] Geoffrey M. Jeffrey, "The Role of Chemotherapy in Malaria Control through Primary Health Care: Constraints and Future Prospects," *Bulletin of the World Health Organization*, vol. 62, supplement (1984), 49–53.

[10] The thirteen countries were Burundi, Central African Republic, Congo, Guinea, Ivory Coast, Lesotho, Liberia, Malawi, Nigeria, Rwanda, Swaziland, Togo, and Zaire. US Department of Health and Human Services, Public Health Service, Centers for Disease

mortality due to malaria, diarrhea, and vaccine-preventable diseases. Tactical Variant I was at the heart of this malaria initiative. Its control strategy relied on the use of drugs, and the CCCD encouraged the creation of national malaria control units. In eleven of the twelve countries that were endemic for malaria, new units were created to work within the PHC systems.[11] But the African commitment to these malaria control programs was not robust, and, over the course of the 1980s, some programs were completely undone by political violence that broke out in Southern, West, and Central Africa.

NEW ZONES OF VIOLENCE AND POLITICAL CHAOS

By the beginning of the 1980s, the white-ruled apartheid regime in South Africa, with its quasi-colony of South West Africa (now Namibia), was the last standing of the colonial-era regimes. The apartheid regime of South Africa was committed to the repression of the anti-apartheid movement in an all-out effort to forestall the emergence of majority African rule. South Africa was surrounded by newly independent African states whose governments were supportive of the anti-apartheid struggle and were willing to provide havens for anti-apartheid fighters. In retaliation, South Africa aggressively attempted to destabilize the anti-apartheid alliance states. In the areas embroiled in this conflict, it was all but impossible to initiate or maintain malaria control programs.

At the dawn of the 1980s, Southern Africa seemed to be the region most cursed by conflict. Soon, however, political disorder struck other areas of the continent. In 1980, a military coup overthrew the Americo-Liberian government and, within a few years, Liberia was embroiled in war. The civil conflicts continued until a peace agreement was reached in 2003. Approximately 250,000 people died during the conflict. Sierra Leone was embroiled in civil war from 1991 to 2002; approximately 75,000 people lost their lives, and 2 million fled to neighboring countries. A military coup in Sudan in 1989 ushered in a series of wars in the south

Control, International Health Program Office, *Addressing the Challenges of Malaria Control in Africa* (Washington, D.C.: USAID, Africa Regional Project (698–0421), n.d. [c. 1994]) and US Department of Health and Human Services, Public Health Service, Centers for Disease Control, International Health Program Office, *Controlling Malaria in Africa: Progress and Priorities* (Washington, DC: USAID, Africa Regional Project (698–0421), n.d. [c. 1994].
[11] J. G. Bremen and C. C. Campbell, "Combating Severe Malaria in African Children," *Bulletin of the World Health Organization*, vol. 66, no. 5 (1988), 611–620.

and west of that country. Hundreds of thousands of people lost their lives, and millions were turned into refugees.

But by far the largest, longest, and most destructive conflict took place in the heart of central Africa. The murderous, episodic ethnic pogroms launched between Tutsi and Hutu communities in Rwanda and Burundi since 1959 morphed into large-scale genocide in 1994, when approximately 800,000 people, mostly Tutsi, were hacked to death with machetes in Rwanda. When an invading Tutsi military force ousted the Hutu government, a massive exodus of Rwandans – mostly Hutu – flooded into Zaire (now Democratic Republic of Congo). This further destabilized eastern Zaire, and when neighboring states became involved in the chaos in an effort to unseat Zaire's President Mobutu, the central African region descended into a nightmare of butchery. To date, more than 5 million people have lost their lives.[12]

The overall significance of these conflicts for malaria control was bleak. Malaria control was barely possible: the war zones incubated a range of infections because refugees were generally malnourished, without recourse to basic sanitation or clean water, and often slept in makeshift shelters exposed to mosquitoes and other insects.

POPULATION GROWTH AND ECOLOGICAL CHANGE

Beyond the zones of conflict, in the rest of rural and urban tropical Africa, other forces were transforming the distribution of malarial infections. One of the most important – arguably the most important – was population growth. The rates of population increase in sub-Saharan Africa were among the highest in the world during the postcolonial period. Over the period 1950–2001, sub-Saharan populations grew at an average rate of 2.6 percent per year.[13]

---

[12] For an introduction to the conflicts, see Jason K. Stearns, *Dancing in the Glory of Monsters: The Collapse of the Congo and the Great War of Africa* (New York: Public Affairs, 2011).

[13] Benno J. Ndulu and Stephen A. O'Connell, "Policy Plus," table 1.4 Long-Run Growth Rates of Regional Population, GDP, and GDP Per Capita, 16.

  Many African states lacked the technical capacity and/or the political interest to gather reliable population data. For African population estimates drawn from data available online from the International Programs Center of the US Bureau of the Census, available online: http://www.census.gov/population/international, see Angus Maddison, *The World Economy: Historical Statistics* (Paris: OECD [Development Centre of the Organisation for Economic Co-operation and Development, 2003]), 201–208.

This robust growth accelerated population movements that extended two earlier patterns. The first was rural–urban migration. It continued apace, and urban populations grew more rapidly than ever. This had the effect of reducing the level of exposure to endemic malaria infection and reducing the burden of malaria for urban populations in comparison to rural populations.

The second pattern was the expansion of rural populations into new lands. Rural population growth meant that villagers who remained in the countryside converted new lands to agriculture by dint of necessity. This was true across all biomes, and in some areas the ecological transformations were extensive. In the savanna regions, villagers developed new rice fields along the floodplains of rivers. In the drylands, they opened up new fields for peanut, maize, sorghum, and millet. In the more humid woodlands, they expanded the cultivation of cocoa and cassava. Some of the biome conversions were endorsed by the state, as in the "Terres Neuves" colonization program in Senegal that attempted to organize and regulate settler movements. In most states, however, movements to new lands advanced principally through the initiative of pioneers who moved their families and undertook the arduous work of clearing savanna and open woodlands and preparing the soils.

The most humid biomes also attracted newcomers. Villagers expanded their agricultural settlements into the West and Central African rainforests. Particularly in the coastal zones, timber companies also rushed in to digest the ecological wealth. They felled giant trees mechanically, and, once cleared, the exposed soils proved shallow and fragile. Financial rewards from the unregulated harvesting of this timber drove high rates of tropical deforestation in a new and accelerated chapter of one of the oldest processes of anthropogenic environmental change in world history.

The international demand for timber transformed the distribution of vector mosquitoes. Deforestation reduced the woodland habitat for *Anopheles funestus* and expanded the habitat for *An. gambiae s.s.* and other species in the *An. gambiae* complex. Malaria transmission in the zones of deforestation went unmeasured, in part because much of the activity was unsanctioned by the state and because timber cutting and hauling involved mobile teams of workers. Once deforested, the lands attracted migrants of modest means who sought to make a living on these thin soils.

Some ecological zones were slated for large-scale capital investment, particularly for rice projects that were designed with the goal of increasing African food production and reducing dependence on food imports. Somewhat surprisingly, the creation of rice fields led to an increase in mosquito density, but generally not to an increase in malaria. The creation of rice fields in Mali, for example, created new mosquito habitat, but the levels of transmission in the irrigated zones were low compared to the nonirrigated zones.[14] Similarly, the creation of rice fields in Kenya provided new breeding grounds, but most mosquitoes took their blood meals from local cattle rather than from human beings, and the incidence of malaria there dropped.[15] This was the so-called *paddies paradox*. The investments in new rice fields typically cleared out *An. funestus*, and in some settings, the colonizing *An. gambiae s.l.* were less efficient transmitters of malaria. In addition, in some settings, participants in these rice projects improved their economic circumstances and thus were able to have better access to health care; many slept under bed nets.[16]

The impacts of biome conversion for agriculture and timbering on malaria transmission were complex and not fully predictable because the prospects for malaria transmission depended on local ecological conditions. Most of the new communities' experiences with malaria went unmonitored during the 1980s and much of the 1990s.

CHLOROQUINE RESISTANCE IN TROPICAL AFRICA

Resistance to chloroquine developed early in the era of the global malaria eradication campaign. In 1957, researchers noted the first cluster of falciparum parasites resistant to the wonder drug along the Thai–Cambodian border, and the resistance spread quickly into Thailand. A few years later, in 1960, two separate clusters emerged in South America, in Venezuela and Colombia. Yet another focus of resistance was reported in Papua New Guinea in 1976.

In tropical Africa, chloroquine-resistant falciparum malaria first appeared in 1978 in nonimmune travelers who had visited Kenya and Tanzania, and within a few years there were more reports of resistance in

---

[14] Guimogo Dolo, Lolivier J.T. Briët, Adama Dao, Sékou F. Traoré, Madama Bouaré, Nafomon Sogoba, Oumou Niaré, Magaran Bagayogo, Djibril Sangaré, Thomas Teuscher, and Yeya T. Touré, "Malaria Transmission in Relation to Rice Cultivation in the Irrigated Sahel of Mali," *Acta Tropica*, vol. 89, no. 2 (2004), 147–159.

[15] C.M. Mutero, C. Kabutha, V. Kimani, L. Kabuage, G. Gitau, J. Ssennyonga, J. Githure, L. Muthami, A. Kaida, L. Musyoka, E. Kiarie, and M. Oganda, "A Transdisciplinary Perspective on the Links between Malaria and Agroecosystems in Kenya," *Acta Tropica*, vol. 89, no. 2 (2004), 171–186.

[16] J.N. Ijumba and S.W. Lindsay, "Impact of Irrigation on Malaria in Africa: Paddies Paradox," *Medical and Veterinary Entomology*, vol. 15, no. 1 (2001), 1–11.

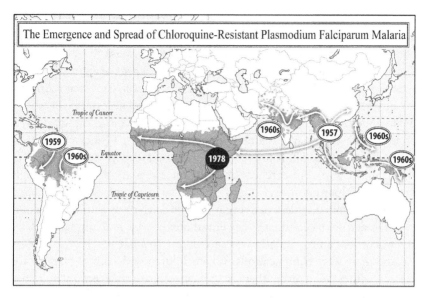

MAP 5.2. The Emergence and Spread of Chloroquine-Resistant Plasmodium Falciparum Malaria
Adapted from: Andreas Ecker, Adele M. Lehane, Jérôme Clain, and David A. Fidock. "PfCRT and Its Role in Antimalarial Drug Resistance," *Trends in Parasitology*, vol. 28, no. 11 (2012), 505.

Madagascar, Tanzania, and Kenya. By 1983, resistance had spread from the East African coastal areas into Sudan, Uganda, Zambia, and Malawi. Genetic studies indicated that the parasite resistance could be traced back to Southeast Asia.[17] By 1988, chloroquine resistance had reached every country in tropical Africa.[18] See Map 5.2.

Chloroquine resistance only slowly became a major problem. At first, chloroquine was fully effective against most falciparum infections and remained the front-line drug of treatment. Gradually, however, the number of treatment failures grew, and the tragedies from clinical malaria began to climb. The first longitudinal study took place in Senegal. There, malaria researchers had studied three rural populations in different ecological zones – the sahel, savanna, and forest – before the emergence of

[17] A. O. Talisuna, P. Bloland, and U. D'Alessandro, "History, Dynamics, and Public Health Importance of Malaria Parasite Resistance," *Clinical Microbiology Reviews*, vol. 17, no. 1 (2004), 236–237.
[18] Jean-François Trape, "The Public Health Impact of Chloroquine Resistance in Africa," *American Journal of Tropical Medicine and Hygiene*, vol. 64, nos. 1–2 (2001), 12–17.

chloroquine resistance in 1990. They continued their observations for another five years, until 1995. Deaths had increased dramatically among children, ranging from a two-fold to eleven-fold increase.[19]

Deaths from malaria soared to levels not seen since the colonial period. After agonizing delays, medical personnel succeeded in convincing African governments that new treatment protocols were necessary. In 1993, Malawi became the first African country to switch from chloroquine to a combination drug, sulfadoxine-pyrimethamine (SP). Clinicians in other countries also tried SP. It proved to be a useful stopgap measure, but, by 1994, in Tanzania, researchers in a therapeutic study discovered a high level of falciparum resistance to SP.[20] The genie of resistance, once unleashed, ripped a destructive path through the populations of small children across the continent. The era of inexpensive and efficacious drug treatment for clinical malaria was shuddering to a halt.

And there were complications. When children with clinical malaria are treated with a failing drug, there is an increased risk of severe anemia. In a hospital setting, this condition can be treated with blood transfusions. But, by the early 1990s, many blood supplies were tainted with the human immunodeficiency virus (HIV), and in some countries, tainted blood supplies are thought to have accounted for approximately one-quarter of HIV infections in children.[21]

The welling failure of chloroquine sparked a surge of interest in African plant products that might be useful as mosquito repellents. In Guinea Bissau, for example, Western researchers discovered that Africans burned a number of different plants, both outdoors and indoors, to reduce mosquito biting activity and that all but one had a significant impact on mosquito activity. Some of the same plants produced oils that could be

---

[19] Jean-François Trape, Gilles Pison, Marie-Pierre Preziosi, Catherine Enel, Annabel Desgrées du Loû, Valérie Delaunay, Badara Samb, Emmanuel Lagarde, Jean-François Molez, and François Simondon, "Impact of Chloroquine Resistance on Malaria Mortality," *Comptes rendus de l'Académie des Sciences*, vol. 321, no. 8 (1998), 689–697.

[20] A. M. Rønn, H. A. Msangeni, J. Mhina, W. H. Wernsdorfer, and I. C. Bygbjerg, "High Level of Resistance of *Plasmodium falciparum* to Sulfadoxine-Pyrimethamine in Children in Tanzania," *Transactions of the Royal Society of Tropical Medicine and Hygiene*, vol. 90, no. 2 (1996), 179–181.

[21] Talisuna et al., "History, Dynamics, and Public Health Importance," 247, citing Nathan Shaffer, Katrina Hedberg, Farzin Davachi, Bongo Lyamba, Joel G. Breman, Odette Samu Masisa, Frieda Behets, Allen Hightower, and Phuc Nguyen-Dinh, "Trends and Risk Factors for HIV-1 Seropositivity among Outpatient Children, Kinshasa, Zaire," *AIDS*, vol. 4, no. 12 (1990): 1231–1236.

On the broader historical context of blood transfusion in Africa, see Schneider, *A History of Blood Transfusion in Sub-Saharan Africa*.

applied to the skin; these, too, reduced the number of mosquito bites that users received.[22] Yet these were "traditional" practices that, although they might have reduced nuisance mosquito bites and the number of bites from infected anopheline mosquitoes, did not seem to have any discernible impact on various malariometric indices.[23]

Another surge of interest was directed toward plants thought to have antimalarial properties that Africans used to reduce the suffering from malaria. One of the most promising was the neem tree (*Azadirachta indica*), native to South and Southeast Asia.[24] The National Academy Press published a volume entitled *Neem: A Tree for Solving Global Problems* in 1992, and a number of international conferences were held to explore the prospects for a range of useful neem products. But little came of these initiatives as far as malaria control was concerned. The versatility of neem made it appropriate for home treatment, and, in Nigeria, neem tea infusions were used to treat malaria. Neem seed and leaf extracts were shown effective against malaria parasites, including both those that were resistant to chloroquine and those that were sensitive to it, and some researchers called for a drug development program.[25]

Yet Africans continued to use chloroquine throughout most of the subcontinent. Chloroquine was very inexpensive and readily available in small commercial shops, and these small shops were the principal point of access to malaria treatment. Indeed, in the early 1980s, only 20 percent of rural Africans were estimated to have easy access to any kind of medical

---

[22] Katinka Pålsson and Thomas G. T. Jaenson, "Plant Products Used as Mosquito Repellents in Guinea Bissau, West Africa," *Acta Tropica*, vol. 72, no. 1 (1999), 39–52.

[23] Snow et al., "Does Woodsmoke Protect against Malaria?," 449–451.

[24] Many specialists accept that Indian immigrants in the late nineteenth century introduced the neem tree into eastern Africa because of its well-known and widely appreciated medical properties, although I have not found any historical documentation that explicitly supports this claim. In the early twentieth century, the British introduced neem into their colonies in West Africa, in order to supplement the indigenous species with exotics that might have economic uses. [Edward Ayensu, "Plant and Bat Interactions in West Africa," *Annals of the Missouri Botanical Garden*, vol. 61, no. 3 (1974), 713.] By the late twentieth century, the neem tree was found throughout sub-Saharan Africa, its dryland range limited by its modest requirement of rainfall or shallow groundwater.

[25] Biswas et al., "Biological Activities and Medicinal Properties of Neem (*Azadirachta indica*)," 1336–1345. In more recent years, researchers have explored the efficacy of neem as a larvicide that might be used by villagers to suppress mosquito density. See, for example, Rebecca L. Gianotti, Arne Bomblies, Mustafa Dafalla, Ibrahim Issa-Arzika, Jean-Bernard Duchemin, and Elfatih A. B. Eltahir, "Efficacy of Local Neem Extracts for Sustainable Malaria Vector Control in an African Village," *Malaria Journal*, vol. 7 (2008). Available online: http://www.malariajournal.com/content/pdf/1475-2875-7-138.pdf

facilities. Study of the utilization of antimalarials outside of the formal health system was not extensive. A study of communities along the coast of Kenya found that most mothers whose children suffered from malaria sought out antimalarials from commercial shops. A course of treatment of three pills of chloroquine cost the equivalent of nine cents (US) and spared the mother the costs of travel and long waits in line at a medical clinic.[26]

The recourse to chloroquine was part of a larger, changing pattern of seeking treatment for malaria symptoms. A survey of the sparse evidence from eastern, western, central, and southern Africa suggested that most cases of presumed malaria were treated either at home ("self-treatment") or at a clinic. Only a few sufferers sought recourse to local healers. Most efforts to cure began with self-treatment, using either medicines bought in shops or local plant-based medicines. Few, however, used the local remedies as sole treatment. A major shift in African therapeutic practice had taken place in the decades since independence.[27]

TRAGEDIES OF CONTROL-AND-LAPSE

In several regions on the margins of tropical Africa and within tropical Africa, once-successful efforts to control malaria transmission were allowed to lapse. In the 1980s, a confluence of events created a public health disaster in the highlands of Madagascar. The long-term context of this devastating malaria epidemic was sketched out by malariologists at the Institut Pasteur in Madagascar, in a retrospective analysis.

The island of Madagascar had long had two distinct ethnic populations. One was of Malayo-Polynesian origins, centered in the central highlands. Along the island littoral were immigrants from mainland sub-Saharan Africa. The highland populations with Malayo-Polynesian ancestry typically did not carry the Duffy antigen negativity mutation that protected against vivax, and it seems likely that they had long been subject to endemic

---

[26] R. W. Snow, N. Peshu, D. Forster, H. Mwenesi, and K. Marsh, "The Role of Shops in the Treatment and Prevention of Childhood Malaria on the Coast of Kenya," *Transactions of the Royal Society of Tropical Medicine and Hygiene*, vol. 86, no. 3 (1992), 237–239.

[27] S. C. McCombie, "Treatment Seeking for Malaria: A Review of Recent Research," *Social Science and Medicine*, vol. 43, no. 6 (1996), 933–945. Another literature survey found that more than three-quarters of the population in many countries took recourse to self-treatment. [U. Brinkmann and A. Brinkman, "Malaria and Health in Africa: The Present Situation and Epidemiological Trends," *Tropical Medicine and Parasitology*, vol. 42 (1991), 207–208.]

vivax infections, particularly those rural villagers who worked in the rice fields that were also the breeding grounds of anopheline mosquitoes. The highland kingdom began to import captives of African descent into the highlands, and it is likely that these captives introduced falciparum there. In 1878, the first documented epidemic of malaria broke out. A second epidemic followed in 1895–1896, at the time of the French colonial conquest. Thereafter, falciparum parasites continued to compete for a niche in the mosaic of infections, and a rough equilibrium of 50 percent vivax and 50 percent falciparum infections became established in the highlands.

Highland malaria for the most part was highly localized, sporadically burdening communities around the rice fields. French missionaries treated many with quinine and worked to stem the progress of malaria during large-scale outbreaks. Beginning in 1949, the French enrolled highland school-age children in a program for malarial prophylaxis with chloroquine, and, in combination with synthetic insecticides, the antimalaria program achieved nearly full success. Malaria was not completely eradicated in the highlands, but infections were reduced to a small number. By 1957, malaria transmission had been reduced to such a low level that it was no longer a significant public health problem.

Control efforts slackened and were cut back progressively in the early 1960s. There was little malarial disease to prevent. Then, in 1975, there was a significant uptick in infections. Nearly 13,000 cases of clinical malaria were recorded, and the following year, in the central province of Antananarivo, there were thirty deaths. At first, the outbreaks remained localized and grew slowly among a population that was immunologically naïve.

In 1977, in Antananarivo province, there were 37,750 clinical cases and 140 deaths. Thereafter, the epidemic spiraled upward, reaching more than 1,600 deaths in 1984 and 1985, doubling to more than 3,000 deaths in 1985, and doubling again to more than 6,500 in 1986, and reaching a peak of 9,584 deaths in 1988. When the data from Fianarantsoa province were added, some researchers estimated the death tolls at 15,000 per year during the four worst years of the epidemic.[28]

The cause of the epidemic was undoubtedly complex. The government of Madagascar had embarked on a socialist program of development during the 1970s and had established health clinics and hospitals in rural

[28] Sixte Blanchy, A. Rakotonjanabelo, G. Ranaivoson, and E. Rajaonarivelo. "Epidémiologie du paludisme sur les hautes terres malgaches depuis 1878," *Cahiers Santé*, vol. 3 (1993), 155–161.

regions. The international economic downturn of the 1970s, however, had hit the island hard. Incomes had dropped by approximately 40 percent. The government of Madagascar had borrowed heavily to finance its program of the nationalization of industry, and, by 1980, the IMF had imposed an austerity program and price reforms. When the epidemic struck, there was a dearth of antimalarial drugs to treat the critically ill.

Yet beneath the swirl of complex and countervailing forces that complicate the analysis of the epidemic lie two fundamental epidemiological facts. The first was that the colonial-era programs had transformed the mix of malaria parasites. Chloroquine is differentially more effective against vivax than falciparum, and the campaign of chloroquine prophylaxis had all but eliminated vivax from the highlands. The second fact was that this chloroquinization program, in combination with the dramatic reduction in malaria transmission that had been achieved through vector control, had created a population nakedly vulnerable to malaria. By the 1970s, most of the people living in the highlands of Madagascar were nonimmune. When the epidemic took hold, this population had no acquired immunities with which to buffer the onslaught. The tragedy of control-and-lapse took the lives of tens of thousands of victims.

The creation of nonimmune populations was, however, one of the unavoidable and integral consequences of successful malaria control, and it was not one restricted to the Madagascar highlands. From 1980 to 1981, a malaria eradication project took place on the islands of São Tomé and Príncipe in the Gulf of Guinea. As had been the case on other small islands, interventionists found that local transmission could be fully interrupted by using synthetic insecticides. Eradication seemed at hand. In 1983, however, migrant fishermen reintroduced falciparum malaria to the islands, and, in 1986, an epidemic broke out. It took more lives during its ten-month resurgence than had died from malaria in the seven years before "eradication."[29]

In Sudan, a third episode of control-and-lapse exploded disastrously in the Gezira-Managil irrigation scheme in the region between the Blue and White Nile Rivers. The region had been a focus of long-standing malaria control because of its high economic importance as the center of cotton production for export and the principal source of state revenues.

[29] J. G. Viegas de Ceita, "Malaria in São Tomé and Príncipe," in A. A. Buck (ed.), *Proceedings of the Conference on Malaria in Africa, Practical Considerations on Malaria Vaccines and Clinical Trials, Washington, D.C., December 1–4, 1986* (Washington, DC: American Institute of Biological Sciences, 1987), 142–155.

Following an epidemic in 1971, project managers launched a program of emergency house-spraying, and malaria was brought under control for several years. Another epidemic broke out in the mid-1970s, and it again was countered with IRS. The spraying with synthetic biocides in the cotton fields and houses produced mosquito resistance to gamma-hexachlorocyclohexane (HCH), dieldrin (DLD), DDT, and malathion.

In 1979, a new health initiative, the Blue Nile Health Project (BNHP), was launched in response to a broad health crisis that included a range of infectious diseases, of which snail-borne bilharzia (schistosomiasis) and malaria were the most dangerous. The project oversaw the extension of IRS into villages at risk and undertook environmental modifications to eliminate vector breeding areas. Other interventions followed, such as canal weeding, the use of fish to consume mosquito larvae, and improved drainage systems. National political turmoil spilled into the project, beginning in 1984, and many of the senior staff members were jailed while others fled the country. Even so, by 1989, health initiatives had been implemented in about half of the entire Gezira-Managil System, reaching about 1 million people.

Then, in 1989, malaria rates quadrupled in the study zone as the BNHP project was winding down. In 1990, heavy rains flooded the drainage systems and increased the density of the vectors that transmitted malaria. No drugs or insecticides were available; donor funding had come to an end. The ten years of work of the BNHP ground to a halt, and malaria tore through the population.[30]

Like the initiative undertaken in the highlands of Madagascar, the "control" of malaria had been a double-edged sword. Protection had been purchased at the expense of immunity. And when protection failed, owing to political upheaval, donor fatigue, or the failure of control technologies, the "protected" populations became newly vulnerable to the ravages of malaria.

For the malariologists who watched in horror at the unraveling of successful control, the lessons were difficult to digest. What were the key variables to maintaining control? Was successful control dependent on internal political stability? If so, this boded poorly for the control of malaria across much of tropical Africa. The entirety of the central African region was in turmoil, and it was unclear when or how political

[30] Jobin, *Dams and Disease*, 335–353.

order would be re-established. Major conflicts continued in Sudan, and in West Africa, some states were failing and warlordism was the rubric for Western understanding of the political chaos that ensued. From this perspective, malaria control programs could not possibly be undertaken on a subcontinent-wide basis. They would necessarily have to be selective national programs, centered on urban areas and economic centers of importance to the states involved.

Other major outbreaks of malaria took place on the highland frontiers of mainland tropical Africa during the 1980s and 1990s. The populations in these areas of unstable infection made up a small percentage of the overall sub-Saharan population, but their vulnerabilities made them epidemiologically significant, and researchers began to investigate the association between increased rainfall and other variables of weather and changes in the density and longevity of the vector mosquitoes. Research linked some of the epidemics to global weather events such as El Niño, yet it was clear that other weather variables, such as temperature fluctuations and local rainfall events, were deeply implicated. Indeed, local conditions and local epidemiology could often be determinative.[31] The impact of these epidemics varied. Some were intensely destructive: between 1995–2000, epidemic malaria in the highlands of western Uganda caused a large increase in under-five mortality at the same time that decreases in under-five mortality were registered in other parts of the country. The increased rate of child mortality in the highlands of western Uganda was so large that when the data were integrated into the national data set, they produced an overall national increase in under-five mortality.[32]

Were ongoing financial commitments from external donors necessary for successful malaria control? If so, during the 1980s and into the mid-1990s, this question was moot. There were no protocols for successful control that could be scaled up, and thus there were no calls for massive and continuing financial commitments.

[31] J. Mouchet, S. Manguin, J. Sircoulon, S. Laventure, O. Faye, A. W. Onapa, P. Carnevale, J. Julvez, and D. Fontenille, "Evolution of Malaria in Africa for the Past 40 Years: Impact of Climatic and Human Factors," *Journal of the American Mosquito Control Association*, vol. 14, no. 2 (1998), 121–130; Kim A. Lindblade, Edward D. Walker, Ambrose W. Onapa, Justus Katungu, and Mark L. Wilson, "Highland Malaria in Uganda: Prospective Analysis of an Epidemic Associated with El Niño," *Transactions of the Royal Society of Tropical Medicine and Hygiene*, vol. 93, no. 5 (1999), 480–487.

[32] Fred Nuwaha, Juliet Babirye, and Natal Ayiga, "Why the Increase in under-Five Mortality in Uganda from 1995 to 2000? A Retrospective Analysis," *BMC Public Health*, vol. 11 (2011), 725. Available online: http://www.biomedcentral.com/1471-2458/11/725

TO IMPROVE THE RATES OF CHILD SURVIVAL

In the mid-1990s, USAID launched a new initiative to improve the survival rates of African children. Two of its constituent parts were a set of guidelines for the treatment of malaria that focused on the recognition and management of acute and chronic malaria and another for the treatment and management of malaria in pregnant women.[33] It also suggested a path that led to the current era of insecticide-treated bed nets to reduce transmission.[34]

USAID undertook clinical studies of the impact of treatment and management of malaria in pregnant women in Malawi. The issue was of high importance because even women who lived in holoendemic areas and who had a robust acquired immunity to malaria infections were likely to lose their immunities during pregnancy. They regained their pre-pregnancy immune status at about the time of delivery. Their vulnerabilities were greatest during first pregnancies, but even during successive pregnancies, many women studied had high levels of parasitemia and placental infections. The USAID findings underscored the medical efficaciousness of using antimalarial drugs to reduce malarial infections in the pregnant woman, her placenta, and the umbilical cord. Children born of treated women had improved birthweight and a lower risk of neonatal and infant mortality. The studies made it clear that an antimalarial drug intervention for high-risk pregnancies should be a part of any malaria control or antenatal care program.[35]

This was the first significant advance in therapeutic approaches to malaria control in the twentieth century and was the harbinger of an approach known as *intermittent preventive therapy* (IPT). It first hinged on the administration of antimalarials to pregnant women (IPTp) and later was extended to infants (IPTi) and children (IPTc). The intermittent

---

[33] The vulnerability of pregnant women to severe malaria had been recognized for some time. In the early 1980s, studies in western Kenya had highlighted the issue. See B. J. Brabin, "An Analysis of Malaria in Pregnancy in Africa," *Bulletin of the World Health Organization*, vol. 61, no. 6 (1983), 1005–1016.

[34] US Department of Health and Human Services, Public Health Service, Centers for Disease Control, International Health Program Office, *Addressing the Challenges of Malaria Control in Africa* (Washington, DC: USAID, Africa Regional Project (698–0421), n.d., [c. 1994]).

[35] US Department of Health and Human Services, Public Health Service, Centers for Disease Control, International Health Program Office, *Malaria Prevention in Pregnancy: The Mangochi Malaria Research Project* (Washington, DC: USAID, Africa Regional Project (698–0421), n.d., [c. 1993]).

treatment of infants and children was found to reduce significantly mortality and morbidity and to improve their general health. The researchers had unknowingly rediscovered the empirical findings of Belgian colonial physicians in the 1930s.

THE SYNERGIES OF HIV/MALARIA INFECTIONS

The first positive case of HIV infection in the world can be dated with some certainty to 1959 in Kinshasa, in the last year of Belgian colonial control. The human virus had originated as a simian virus in western equatorial Africa and had passed from animals to humans at least eleven times and perhaps many more.[36]

The low level infection first flared into an epidemic outbreak of HIV during the 1970s, probably in Kinshasa. As John Iliffe, the outstanding historian of the African acquired immunodeficiency syndrome (AIDS) epidemic, noted: "The world's first HIV epidemic among a heterosexual population had begun before the existence of the virus was even suspected. That, more than anything else, was why Africa was to suffer so terribly during the following decades."[37]

There were two principal strains of the virus, and they both expanded their spheres during the decade of the 1980s. The less virulent HIV-2 infection spread from central Africa into western Africa. HIV-2 killed hundreds of thousands, but it never reached the levels of prevalence of HIV-1. The highly virulent HIV-1 infection spread from central Africa to the east. It was first reported in Uganda in 1982 and in Tanzania in 1983, and from eastern Africa, it spread both north and south. It reached southern Africa in the early 1990s, and there it achieved unprecedented levels of prevalence, becoming the world's worst epidemic of HIV.[38]

The epidemic afflicted a number of different age cohorts. HIV/AIDS struck down children who contracted the virus in utero from their infected mothers. If they survived until birth, they sickened thereafter and rarely lived beyond early childhood. The principal age cohorts afflicted, however, were sexually active young and middle-aged adults, and the tragedy of their deaths produced a broader social catastrophe of millions of orphans,

---

[36] John Iliffe, *The African AIDS Epidemic: A History* (Athens: Ohio University Press, 2006), 3–4.
[37] Iliffe, *African AIDS Epidemic*, 12.
[38] Iliffe, *African AIDS Epidemic*, 19–64.

many of whom lived at the edge of material existence. As the HIV/AIDS epidemic came into focus, its scale and the visibility of the victims' suffering all but immersed the rising wave of malaria deaths. Malaria killed princi- pally small children in rural areas, and there were other childhood afflic- tions, such as diarrheal diseases, that confounded the epidemiological accounting of deaths. The tragedy of HIV/AIDS for a time eclipsed the tragedy of malaria.

It was not until 2005 that researchers documented the terrible synergy between HIV-1 and malaria. Individuals afflicted with HIV-1 were less able to survive the challenges of severe malarial infections. HIV-1 infections caused more malaria deaths by increasing the proportion of severe malaria cases, the case fatality rate for severe infections, and the failure rate of antimalarial therapy.[39] Across all of sub-Saharan Africa, the HIV-1 epi- demic was estimated to have increased malaria deaths by 4.9 percent, with most of the worst impacts concentrated in southern and eastern Africa.[40]

BUILDING CAPACITY FOR MALARIA CONTROL

In response to the unfolding malaria disaster, in 1992 the WHO convened a Ministerial Malaria Conference in Amsterdam. The conference adopted a Global Malaria Control Strategy whose four basic elements called for disease control through early diagnosis and treatment, selective and sus- tainable preventive measures, detection and intervention to contain or prevent epidemics, and the strengthening of capacities to regularly assess the national malaria situation.[41] It was a giant step away from the erad- ication era. The goals for the new control strategy were lofty: to reduce malaria mortality in the year 2000 by 20 percent compared to 1995. By the end of 1996, more than 10,000 individuals were in training at the district and community levels, and by mid-1997, some forty-seven of forty-nine

---

[39] E.L. Korenromp, G. Williams, S.J. de Vlas, E. Gouws, C.F. Gilks, P.D. Ghys, and B.L. Nahlen, "Malaria Attributable to the HIV-1 Epidemic, Sub-Saharan Africa," *Emerging Infectious Diseases*, vol. 11, no. 9 (2005), 1413.

[40] Korenromp et al., "Malaria Attributable to the HIV-1 Epidemic," 1415.

[41] The World Health Assembly in 1993, the Forty-Ninth Session of the United Nations General Assembly and the Thirty-Third Ordinary Session of the Assembly of Heads of State in 1994, and the Government of the Organization of African Unity in 1997 confirmed the Global Malaria Control Strategy. [P.I. Trigg and A.V. Kondrachine, "Commentary: Malaria Control in the 1990s," *Bulletin of the World Health Organization*, vol. 76, no. 1 (1998), 13.]

countries in sub-Saharan Africa had produced national malaria control plans.[42] In 1998, the WHO launched a new program, Roll Back Malaria (RBM), in an effort to coordinate national efforts to reduce malaria morbidity and mortality. In 2000, at a WHO conference in Abuja, Nigeria, African heads of state pledged their support for the goal of reducing malaria deaths by 50 percent by 2010.

The RBM program represented a new and fundamentally different approach to the provision of antimalarial therapy. It shifted the focus from the clinician and health facility to the home and mother. New resources were committed to it. It aimed high, and, like many of the targets for global health, it was meant to be inspirational, to encourage greater effort. There were, however, significant problems with the roll-out of the RBM program. African states were slow to develop national malaria control programs that were in line with RBM requirements, and donor monies were slow to reach these national programs.[43]

An even larger problem was rooted in the weak, underfunded, and understaffed national health systems. The number of doctors and nurses trained to staff the health systems were inadequate to the tasks, and large numbers of African doctors and nurses found employment overseas, where compensation was higher. Overall, sub-Saharan Africa was short hundreds of thousands of physicians and hundreds of thousands of nurses. Training capacity was low, and the ability to retain staff was weak.[44]

NEW APPROACHES TO A MALARIA VACCINE

Malaria vaccine researchers were pursuing a number of apparently promising paths of investigation during the early and mid-1980s. In 1987, a Colombian researcher, M. E. Patarroyo, announced that he had developed the first synthetic malaria vaccine and had succeeded in protecting monkeys from malaria. His vaccine was based on the use of a protective blood stage antigen that triggered an immunogenic response: the body's defense mechanisms were kick-started to provide protection. This was the same general approach that some other labs had taken, but Patarroyo appeared to have brilliantly surmounted some bedeviling obstacles.

---

[42] Trigg and Kondrachine, "Commentary: Malaria Control in the 1990s," 14.

[43] Randall M. Packard, *The Making of a Tropical Disease: A Short History of Malaria* (Baltimore: Johns Hopkins University Press, 2007), 220–227.

[44] Charles Hongoro and Barbara McPake, "How to Bridge the Gap in Human Resources for Health," *Lancet*, vol. 364, 16 October 2004, 1451–1456.

Members of the broader vaccine research community responded variously with enthusiasm, envy, and skepticism as the claims came under closer scrutiny and the Patarroyo vaccine underwent clinical trials beginning in the late 1980s and continuing into the late 1990s. The WHO, the Medical Research Council of the United Kingdom, and the Swiss Tropical Institute backed some of the trials, which were undertaken using human volunteers in Brazil, Colombia, Ecuador, Venezuela, Thailand, Tanzania, and the Gambia. After a heady build-up of expectations and hope, the trials produced disappointingly modest overall results and a lack of efficacy in protecting younger infants. The wider malaria research community's summary judgment was stark: there were no prospects to use the vaccine for malaria control in sub-Saharan Africa.[45]

In the early 1990s, following the Malaria Immunology and Vaccine Research (MIVR) scandals involving fraud and the misappropriation of funds, the US government took a new approach to vaccine research. It sought to identify promising vaccine candidates that could be advanced to clinical trials, and, toward this end, it created the Malaria Vaccine Development Program. This gave a new lease on life to vaccine researchers. One approach was to forge forward with ongoing research on a transmission-blocking vaccine that would produce human antibodies that would prove effective against one of the parasite's developmental blood stages, occurring when it was bathed in human blood within the mosquito's gut. The transmission-blocking vaccines prevented the development of sporozoites in the mosquito, rather than preventing infections in human beings, and thus they were sometimes referred to as "altruistic" vaccines. Vaccinated individuals provided protection to others by preventing the transmission of their own infections to mosquitoes. Similar lines of research moved forward in the United Kingdom and at the Tropical Disease Research center at the WHO.[46]

Yet another approach to a vaccine was to reproduce a protein that occurred on the surface of the sporozoite, known as a circumsporozoite protein (CSP), inject it into a human being, and thereby stimulate an immunological reaction that could protect against infections. By the late 1980s, experiments at GlaxoSmithKline had fused such a protein with a hepatitis virus surface antigen to produce what seemed to be a promising

[45] Sherman, *The Elusive Malaria Vaccine*, 184–187.
[46] On the history of transmission-blocking vaccines, see Irwin S. Sherman, *Magic Bullets to Conquer Malaria: From Quinine to Qinghaosu* (Washington, DC: American Society for Microbiology, 2011), 213–230; and Sherman, *Elusive Malaria Vaccine*, 199–215.

vaccine candidate, known as RTS,S. In 1998, trials in the Gambia indicated that the vaccine acted to provide some modest protection against infection and to weaken the symptoms of those who became infected. Following this success, the Bill and Melinda Gates Foundation agreed to provide US$50 million, and RTS,S vaccine research continued.[47]

---

[47] Sherman, *Magic Bullets to Conquer Malaria*, 230–235. Other approaches, including an attenuated sporozoite vaccine and a liver-stage antigen vaccine, are also in development. (Sherman, *Elusive Malaria Vaccine*, 264–283.)

6

The Campaign for Elimination

At the dawn of the twenty-first century, the explosive growth in human immunodeficiency virus (HIV) infections eerily illuminated the epidemiological chasm between the impoverished majority populations in the "Global South" who suffered from the ravages of infectious diseases and the majority populations of the wealthier industrial and postindustrial states for whom the principal threats to health were from high-calorie diets, lack of physical activity, other lifestyle choices, and genetic inheritance. The HIV pandemic shed light on the resurgence of other infectious diseases that were centered in tropical Africa. Some of these infections were opportunistic. The most severe was the old plague of tuberculosis (TB), which was whipped into a deadly storm by the HIV virus. HIV compromised the immune response to TB, and a massive number of latent cases erupted into active cases. Tubercular infections skyrocketed and became the leading cause of death in sub-Saharan Africa. HIV also compromised the immune response to malaria, and, like TB, malaria thus unleashed ran its course with greater malignancy.

The principal driver of the new global public health movement was the HIV/AIDS epidemic, in part because it struck down adults in their most economically productive years. It grossly distorted the normal epidemiological order, and, for some observers, it portended severe economic dislocation. There had been no comparable impact of infectious disease since the global influenza pandemic of 1918–1919 that killed an estimated 20–100 million people. In South Africa, at the beginning of the twenty-first century, the shocking legalistic denials of antiretroviral medications to HIV-positive Africans highlighted as never before the grotesque health inequalities of the contemporary world. Activists in South Africa, the epicenter of the HIV/AIDS epidemic in sub-Saharan Africa, joined forces with activists in the "Global North" to demand change.

Their rhetoric and activism called forth a new level of engagement. The most visible outcome of a new purposefulness in global health was an effort to target the major infectious diseases that ravaged populations in the Global South: AIDS, TB, and malaria. The creation of the Global Fund in 2002 was the culmination of this process. Many of the world's major nations agreed to contribute on an ongoing basis to a central fund that would aim to lower the burden of infectious disease among the poorest populations. In 2005, President George W. Bush announced the President's Malaria Initiative and allocated monies for malaria control. In 2007, to the surprise of the global public health community, the Bill and Melinda Gates Foundation announced that it was launching a new campaign to eradicate malaria.

These newly available financial resources roused enthusiasm for a massive assault on the fortress of tropical African malaria. The goals were noble, the funding generous, the design a work in progress. The first global malaria eradication campaign of the 1950s and 1960s had largely extinguished interest in the field of malariology, and the eminent mid-twentieth-century malariologists had long since retired and passed on. By the early twenty-first century, few malariologists had broad practical experience in malaria control.

Contemporary malaria experts represented two different domains of expertise. One was medical. It was comprised principally of physicians with extensive experience in malaria treatment whose focus was on reducing deaths among pregnant women, infants, and children. The other domain of expertise was molecular. It was comprised of bench scientists who explored the parasite and mosquito genomes in the hopes of developing effective vaccines or of altering the genetic makeup of the parasites and mosquitoes in order to reduce or eliminate transmission.

These new malaria experts came from diverse backgrounds. From the last few decades of the twentieth century, African physicians and scientists came to play prominent roles in research and worked in tandem with their counterparts from the Global North. Important research centers in tropical Africa, such the Kenya Medical Research Institute, the Malaria Research and Training Center in Mali, and the Ifakara Research Center in Tanzania, received financial support from Europe and North America, and more recently, many smaller African institutions became linked with malaria project partners in the Global North through initiatives such as the International Centers for Excellence in Malaria Research, funded by the US National Institutes of Health.

The economic rationale for the new campaign drew on the same arguments that had buttressed the global malaria eradication program of the 1950s and 1960s. The central thrust was that the economic benefits that would accrue from the elimination of malaria would more than repay the investments. Malaria programs would remove constraints on economic growth that would allow African and other less-developed economies to advance more rapidly. This growth in turn would generate financial resources that could support government institutions.[1]

This rationale was convincing to funders and the administrators of government agencies who were in line to receive large dispensations for programs of malaria control and treatment or for molecular research.[2] It made logical sense in contexts in which malarial infections made people very sick and prevented them from engaging in productive activities. It was less persuasive, however, in contexts in which populations were heavily parasitized and many of the economically productive were largely asymptomatic.[3]

A study of the working capacity of adult Liberian men found that there were no major differences between farmers living in regions of holoendemic malaria transmission and mining company workers living in regions of mesoendemic transmission and no differences between the Liberians and normal Swedish men.[4] This suggested that any projected increase in worker productivity that would result from effective malaria control was overstated. It seemed certain, however, that malaria control would prove a boon to foreign investment. Indeed, it was something of a sine qua non for attracting nonimmune expatriates with specialized skills. Investments in malaria control could help to make tropical Africa safer for overseas investment.

This was consonant with a broader development discourse that held that foreign investments in Africa would produce economic growth there. This was a compelling argument for many foreign investors and economic

---

[1] Jeffrey Sachs and Pia Malaney, "The Economic and Social Burden of Malaria," *Nature*, vol. 415, 7 February 2002, 680–685.

[2] On the emerging postwar literature that held that malaria control would produce economic development and the refinements of the early twentieth century, see Packard, "'Roll Back Malaria, Roll in Development?,'" 53–87.

[3] Interestingly, there was no effort to determine the economic impact of malaria control that had been achieved through the African-initiated use of chloroquine. It was as though the successful intervention had never taken place.

[4] J. Brohult et al., "The Working Capacity of Liberian Males: A Comparison between Urban and Rural Populations in Relation to Malaria," *American Journal of Tropical Medicine and Parasitology*, vol. 75, no. 5 (1981), 487–494.

development theoreticians; it was less so for those who had witnessed the corruption engendered by capital investments in the extractive industries of precious metals, rare earths, and oil mining. In the postcolonial period, these extractive industries often generated disenfranchisement and squalor and left behind desperate poverty. Most of these industrial profits fled Africa.

There were other problematic dimensions to the discourse that was mobilized to support the new eradication initiative. Some authors claimed that Africans had been excluded from the global malaria eradication program of the mid-twentieth century and argued that this could be ascribed to neglect, colonial-era racism, or scarcity of resources. Now Africa's turn had come. The administrators of a welter of nongovernmental organizations (NGOs) and government agencies rushed to apprize themselves of basic malariology. The machinery for a major public health intervention was thrown into gear. There was enormous good that could be done. How should the malaria control programs proceed? Could the good be sustained?

Sir Richard Feacham, director of the Global Fund, proposed a two-front global plan for malaria eradication that would begin with control efforts in the environments with the highest levels of transmission, while other countries at the edges of the high transmission environments would work toward eradication. This approach was later conceptualized as "shrinking the malaria map."[5] The initial African forecast was for successful eradication along the southern frontiers of Botswana, Namibia, South Africa, and Swaziland. Eradication would, at a later point, roll north across the continent, consolidating the early gains that had been made in the regions of high transmission and thus liberating Africans from the scourge of malaria.[6] The vision seemed to run counter to the long experience with malaria control in tropical Africa. But the large sums of money pouring into malaria control all but silenced the voices of skeptics. Who could say for sure what would be the impact of a truly massive infusion of money and the organization of collective effort? Who could gainsay an important global public health initiative that would certainly do great good in the short and perhaps the medium term?

[5] Richard G. A. Feacham, Allison A. Phillips, and Geoffrey A. Targett (eds.), *Shrinking the Malaria Map: A Prospectus for Malaria Elimination* (San Francisco: The Global Health Group, 2009).

[6] Richard Feacham and Oliver Sabot, "A New Global Malaria Eradication Strategy," *The Lancet*, vol. 371 (2008) 1633–1635.

BED NETS: RHETORIC AND REALITY

New monies were made available for a massive distribution of bed nets to Africans. Studies conducted in the Gambia in the 1980s had demonstrated that the use of insecticide-treated bed nets (ITNs) could dramatically reduce the toll of malaria, and the hope was that these successes could be replicated across the continent.[7] The historical experience with untreated bed nets, however, suggested that there would be limits to their acceptance and use. Although bed nets had been one of the quintessential protections for white nonimmunes, a substantial percentage of whites had in the past rejected their use because they found that sleeping under a bed net was simply too hot to bear. Historical experience also suggested that the untreated nets tore easily and that the nets frequently trapped mosquitoes inside, where they could be found engorged in the morning. Yet there seemed little doubt that a bed net could be a very important weapon in the public health arsenal. A bed net was relatively inexpensive, and if properly used and in good repair, it could reduce to a small number the nocturnal mosquito bites received in the hours under the net. The bed net seemed to its advocates to be a practical intervention with considerable promise.

A number of assumptions about people, parasites, and mosquitoes underlay the bed net initiative. For bed nets to be highly effective, people needed to sleep under them during the hours in which the female anopheline mosquitoes took their blood meals. But the hours at which African adults and children took to bed varied greatly, as is the case across the globe. Many adults went to sleep long after sundown, often several hours after the vector mosquitoes began to actively seek blood meals. If children and infants went under the bed nets earlier, they would have greater protection. In many rural and urban areas, the temperatures even late at night were oppressive. Bed nets slowed or stopped the flow of air and made nights under the nets even hotter than they would have been otherwise. Many rural Africans made a practice of sleeping outdoors on hot nights.

The bed nets, when put into service, worked quite effectively when they were hung from a hook and when the nets could be tucked in securely under a mat or mattress or could be made to lay flat on the ground to seal off mosquito access. In practice, this was hard to achieve. Mosquitoes

---

[7] U. D'Alessandro, B. Olaleye, P. Langerock, M. K. Aikins, M. C. Thomson, M. K. Cham, B. M. Greenwood, W. McGuire, S. Bennett, M. K. Cham, and B. A. Cham, "Mortality and Morbidity from Malaria in Gambian Children after Introduction of an Impregnated Bednet Programme," *The Lancet*, vol. 345, no. 8948, 25 February 1995, 479–483.

made their way under the nets before they could be secured, and they slipped under when the nets did not lay flat on the ground or when small holes opened up in them. Mosquitoes sought blood meals from an arm, leg, hand, or foot that rested up against the net at some point during the night. Mosquitoes alighted on the nets and made their ways toward the slightly increased air currents that escaped from holes in the net.

The hope for a large reduction in the number of infective bites hinged on the simple idea of treating the mosquito nets with insecticide. If mosquitoes alighted on the ITNs, they might pick up enough insecticide to kill them before they completed a new cycle of parasite development, be irritated by the insecticide and inhibited from biting, or simply repelled. People sleeping under ITNs would act as bait, and many mosquitoes would pick up a deadly dose of insecticide while searching out a blood meal. Bed nets would thus work to reduce the number of infected mosquitoes. As with many epidemiological phenomena, the intervention would work best when a large number of households used ITNs. It was in this sense a community health program.

The rates of bed net efficacy in controlled trials varied. In areas with high rates of infective bites, the bed nets were less efficacious in reducing deaths and severe illness than in areas with low rates. But even in the areas with high rates, the increases in childhood survival and the reductions in severe illness were impressive. A meta-study that assessed the impact of twenty-two trials found that bed net use in the controlled trials reduced childhood mortality by about 20 percent.[8] This was a substantial impact, and advocates began to push for a massive increase in bed net use across Africa. The hope was that the ITN could insinuate itself into rural and urban cultures to produce a lasting and progressive improvement in public health.

The bed net initiative, however, soon encountered political controversy. At what price should bed nets be sold? Or, should the bed nets be subsidized? During the early years of President George W. Bush's first term of office, the advocates for free-market sales of bed nets held the day. The sales model was energized with an enthusiasm for the development of products that would appeal to African consumers. The hope was that the bed net program would thereby become self-financing: the profits from bed net sales would be reinvested to ramp up production.

A core problem was that a bed net cost the equivalent of between US$3 and US$10, and an outlay of this magnitude was beyond the means of the

---

[8] Christian Lengeler, "Insecticide-Treated Bed Nets and Curtains for Malaria Control," *Cochrane Database of Systematic Reviews*, issue 2 (2004), 10.

African poor. Were bed nets to be a privilege of Africans living above the poverty line? If the market restricted access to bed nets of those most in need, would the reduced bed net coverage compromise community health benefits?

A study conducted in highland Kenya laid out the issues squarely. Most of the villagers wanted to purchase bed nets but lacked the financial means to do so.[9] The imposition of fees to recover costs would compromise access to a basic public health good. The authors proposed a radical solution: the subsidization of bed nets for all. That same year, a group of public health specialists laid out the case for an all-Africa free net program. Bed nets should be considered as comparable to vaccination; and, indeed, the mortality and morbidity gains from bed nets were roughly equivalent to the widely successful measles vaccination program in Africa.[10]

The arguments for cost recovery were convincing, too. It was clear from a national study in Tanzania that the sale of bed nets could produce a high rate of coverage, and the revenues could help to finance the ongoing production and distribution of nets. This held the prospect for a new African-based intervention in public health that would be self-sustaining and would improve public health. The downside was that the very poor would not be able to afford a bed net. How should this problem be addressed?

A core question was the optimal trade-off between sustainability and equity. If the sustainability of a bed net program was based on the recovery of costs, it might be possible to provide subsidies to the poor. This approach was tried in a number of states with mixed results. The programs did extend access to a larger swath of the population, and yet only fully subsidized bed nets reached the very poor.

The issue was rendered moot after a flood of financial support became available through the Global Fund and the US President's Malaria Initiative, and concerns about the sustainability of the program moved to the back burner. Bed nets became available in truly astounding quantities, and programs of free net distribution began across the continent. Major

---

[9] H. L. Guyatt, Sam A. Ocholo, and Robert W. Snow, "Too Poor to Pay: Charging for Insecticide Treated Bed Nets in Highland Kenya," *Tropical Medicine and International Health*, vol. 7, no. 10 (2002), 846–850.

[10] Christopher Curtis, Caroline Maxwell, Martha Lemnge, W. L. Kilama, Richard W. Steketee, William A. Hawley, Yves Bergevin, Carlos C. Campbell, Jeffrey Sachs, Awash Teklehaimanot, Sam Ochola, Helen Guyatt, and Robert W. Snow, "Scaling-up Coverage with Insecticide-Treated Nets against Malaria in Africa: Who Should Pay?," *The Lancet Infectious Diseases*, vol. 3, no. 5 (2002), 304–307.

issues with the nets, however, had been little investigated, and they were directly related to the core issue of sustainability.

How long would the bed nets last? The nets were initially estimated to have a useful life of five years. In practice, they were found to last two to three years, and estimates of the projected recurrent costs skyrocketed. It was known that the nets would deteriorate as a result of washing and the wear-and-tear of putting them up nightly; when holes formed, mosquitoes would fly in and take blood meals, sometimes without picking up a dose of insecticide. One solution was to patch them. But sewing closed the holes strained the netting and caused other holes to open up. An advance was made with the development of sturdier netting that had greater structural integrity. But the improved nets still got some holes, still had to be patched regularly, and were still only functional for about two or three years before they had to be replaced.

An even more significant issue was that of the insecticide. It was critically important because either it killed the mosquito right away or shortened its life to the extent that the malaria parasite was unable to complete its life cycle in the mosquito's gut. The only class of insecticides approved for use on the nets was pyrethroids. The other synthetic insecticides were deemed too dangerous for continuous human exposure and direct bodily contact.

From the beginning of the bed net program, it was known that an extensive use of ITNs would produce selection pressure on the mosquitoes and that resistance to the pyrethroids would emerge and spread. It was basic biology. Resistance had been observed Benin, Botswana, Burkina Faso, Ivory Coast, and Senegal in the late 1990s, and calls had been issued for monitoring the situation, even before the roll out of the large program began.[11] Inevitably, as the ITNs and the long-lasting insecticide-treated nets (LLINs) reached more communities and won wider acceptance, resistance emerged as a major threat to malaria control.[12] It was, of course, possible that a new class of insecticides might be developed that would extend the effectiveness of the bed nets until resistance to the new class developed. But this was, for the moment, more or less a theoretical issue. No new insecticide for use on or near sleeping human beings was in the pipeline.

[11] F. Chandre, F. Darier, L. Manga, M. Akogbeto, O. Faye, J. Mouchet, and P. Guillet, "Status of Pyrethroid Resistance in *Anopheles gambiae sensu lato*," *Bulletin of the World Health Organization*, vol. 77, no. 3 (1999), 230–234.

[12] Alex Asidi, Raphael N'Guessen, Martin Akogbeto, Chris Curtis, and Mark Rowland, "Loss of Household Protection from Insecticide-Treated Nets against Pyrethroid-Resistant Mosquitoes, Benin," *Emerging Infectious Diseases*, vol. 18, no. 7 (2012), 1101–1106.

It was perhaps inevitable that a free good such as a bed net would be put to purposes other than those intended by the interventionists. Some uses were strictly utilitarian: for example, a bed net might be twisted into a rope to restrain livestock or unfurled to secure loose items being transported on the top of a bus. Other uses were aesthetic: the colorful bed nets could be fashioned for personal adornment or wedding gowns. Some uses had unintended consequences. Some of the nets were used to catch fish – a major source of protein for many African communities; in water, the nets lost their insecticidal coatings, although the concentrations of released pyrethroids were deemed by the WHO to be too low to constitute a toxic threat to the fish. Because the nets caught the smallest fish, however, they could significantly compromise piscine resources.

INDOOR RESIDUAL SPRAYING

The other major vector control technique was IRS with synthetic insecticides. As with bed nets, the rationale for control was based on the understanding that the various malaria-transmitting species had fixed patterns of behavior that the malaria control specialists could exploit. One critically important working assumption was that the major anopheline vectors took their blood meals indoors.[13] Researchers, however, soon began to document that the IRS interventions changed the population mix of the vectors. IRS in western Kenya, for example, killed large numbers of *Anopheles gambiae s.s.* that fed indoors. It killed far fewer *An. arabiensis*, which took blood meals both indoors and outdoors, and thus shifted the balance toward outdoor biting.[14] In the sahel of Burkina Faso, a new subspecies of anopheline mosquito was discovered that seemed to be more purely "outdoor biting."[15]

---

[13] The Garki project of the 1970s had demonstrated the critical importance of outdoor biting. See Molineaux and Gramiccia, *The Garki Project*, 290–292.

[14] M. Nabie Bayoh, Derrick K. Mathias, Maurice R. Odiere, Francis M. Mutuku, Luna Kamau, John E. Gimnig, John M. Vulule, William A. Hawley, Mary J. Hamel, and Edward D. Walker, "*Anopheles gambie*: Historical Population Decline Associated with Regional Distribution of Insecticide-Treated Bed Nets in Western Nyanza Province, Kenya," *Malaria Journal*, vol. 9, no. 62 (2010). Available online: http://www.malaria-journal.com/content/9/1/62

[15] Michelle M. Riehle, Wamdaogo M. Guelbeogo, Awa Gneme, Karin Eiglmeier, Inge Holm, Emmanuel Bischoff, Thierry Garnier, Gregory M. Snyder, Xuanzhong Li, Kyriacos Markianos, N'Fale Sagnon, and Kenneth D. Vernick, "A Cryptic Subgroup of *Anopheles gambiae* Is Highly Susceptible to Human Malaria Parasites," *Science*, vol. 331, 4 February 2011, 596–598.

The Roll Back Malaria program stressed ITNs in its early years, but in 2001, the WHO added IRS programs to the arsenal of integrated vector management (IVM) programs. Several African states adopted the WHO IVM ideas and, with assistance from the Global Fund, began to spray houses with insecticides, linking such spraying with bed net use where possible. In Zambia, for example, teams of sprayers covered the insides of houses with insecticides in five regions in which the levels of ITN use were high. The overall results were very positive: as bed net use increased and the number of people sleeping in sprayed houses increased, the levels of morbidity and mortality dropped sharply. As had been the case during the era of the malaria eradication programs of the 1950s and 1960s, it was possible to achieve remarkable levels of control, and, in those regions where the interventions took place, remarkable declines in transmission.[16]

Similar experiences unfolded in several other African countries. The combination of indoor spraying with bed net use was powerful. Benin saw major reductions. In the heady years from 2005–2010, significant reductions began to be recorded across tropical Africa, outside of the war zones in central Africa. Even some of the recently war-torn West African states such as Sierra Leone and Liberia were thought to be candidates for malaria control.

As in the global malaria eradication program of the mid-twentieth century, however, malaria teams found that it was not possible to reduce levels of transmission to zero and that most of the gains in reduced mortality and morbidity came in the first years of the programs. Thereafter, resistance to the insecticides began to develop. The insecticides worked by killing mosquitoes that alighted on the sprayed interior walls. If the mosquitoes died shortly after exposure, they fell to the floor. Researchers could count the dead mosquitoes and calculate the killing effectiveness of the insecticides; this is known as the "knockdown rate." They discovered that surviving mosquitoes had a gene that made them less susceptible to the insecticides. This was dubbed the *knockdown resistance* or kdr gene. Many mosquitoes with the kdr gene lived to reproduce, and, in short order, the kdr gene became predominant in areas with heavy spray coverage. In Zambia, after early dramatic successes during the malaria "elimination"

---

[16] Emmanuel Chanda, Fred Masaninga, Michael Coleman, Chadwick Sikaala, Cecilia Katebe, Michael MacDonald, Kumar S Baboo, John Govere, and Lucien Manga, "Integrated Vector Management: The Zambian Experience," *Malaria Journal*, vol. 7 (2008), no. 194. Available online: http://www.malariajournal.com/content/pdf/1475-2875-7-164.pdf

era, researchers detected high levels of mosquito resistance to pyrethroids and DDT. By 2010, mortality and morbidity rates had begun to rise, although they were far below preintervention levels.[17]

This, too, was a replay of the experience of the 1950s and 1960s, when DDT resistance had emerged rapidly in western Africa and only slowly, if at all, in eastern Africa. In the earlier eradication campaign, the spraying programs had shifted to the other organochlorines, dieldrin (DLD) and benzene hexachloride (BHC), which had higher toxicities than DDT. Fortunately, there were four classes of insecticides that could be deployed in the second eradication campaign: the organochlorine DDT, organophosphates (known as OPs), carbamates, and pyrethroids.

In West Africa, the kdr gene was still in circulation in the vector mosquitoes in the early twenty-first century, and it spread rapidly once again under the pressure of DDT use. The pyrethroids were deployed sparingly for indoor spraying because it was feared that their wider adoption, in combination with their use on bed nets, would accelerate the emergence of resistance and might bring an early demise to the bed net era. Yet resistance to the pyrethroids developed widely.[18] In Benin, where resistance to the pyrethroids and DDT was widespread, the insecticide bendiocarb (a carbamate) was the next line of defense. Carbamates were more expensive than DDT, and they, too, were initially highly effective.[19] But it was only a matter of time before they, too, began to select for resistance more broadly. One hope was that it might be possible to switch between classes of insecticides to slow down the emergence of resistance. The spraying programs continued to forge forward, saving lives and preventing infections, without an endgame in view. IRS would grow both more expensive and less effective over time.

---

[17] Emmanuel Chanda, Janet Hemingway, Immo Kleinschmidt, Andrea M. Rehman, Varsha Ramdeen, Faustina N. Phiri, Sarel Coetzer, David Mthembu, Cecelia J. Shinondo, Elizabeth Chizema-Kawesha, Mulakwa Kamuliwo, Victor Mukonka, Kumar S. Baboo, and Michael Coleman, "Insecticide Resistance and the Future of Malaria Control in Zambia," *PLOS ONE*, vol. 6, no. 9 (2011), 1–9.

[18] Hilary Ranson, Raphael N'Guessan, Jonathan Lines, Nicolas Moiroux, Zinga Nkuni, Vincent Corbel, "Pyrethroid Resistance in African Anopheline Mosquitoes: What Are the Implications for Malaria Control?," *Trends in Parasitology*, vol. 27, no. 2 (2011), 91–98.

[19] G. G. Padonou, M. Sezonlin, R. Ossé, N. Aizoun, F. Oké-Agbo, O. Oussou, G. Gbédjissi, and M. Akogbéto, "Impact of Three Years of Large Scale Indoor Residual Spraying (IRS) and Insecticide Treated Nets (ITNs) Interventions on Insecticide Resistance in *Anopheles gambiae s. l.* in Benin," *Parasites and Vectors*, vol. 5, issue, 1, no. 72 (2012). Available online: http://www.parasitesandvectors.com/content/pdf/1756-3305-5-72.pdf

The reasons for the enthusiastic commitment to large-scale IRS in tropical Africa remained something of a mystery. Its record in tropical Africa, even if only imperfectly known, was not encouraging. Such enthusiasm might be attributed, in part, to a triumph of hope over experience. Another line of explanation might be found in the historical record of IRS in Central and South America, which was, on balance, more positive than in tropical Africa, in that DDT had been used for a more extended period without producing major vector resistance. Some of its most vociferous advocates projected the benefits of the extensive use of DDT in tropical Africa on the basis of the experience in the Americas.[20]

Some advocacy groups threw their support behind the use of DDT and used the occasion to put forward the claim that environmentalist groups had succeeded in banning the use of DDT for malaria control and, as a result, had taken the lives of countless millions of Africans. In the claims were elements of truth intertwined with inaccuracies and misstatements of fact. DDT had fallen out of use in most of West Africa in the 1960s because it produced resistance, not because it had been banned. The major successes in malaria control during the 1960s and 1970s had come about through the broad availability and low cost of chloroquine. Environmentalist groups had attempted to apply pressure to abandon the use of DDT, but there had been no broad interest on the part of African governments to fund IRS programs during the long decades before the creation of the Roll Back Malaria program, the Global Fund, and the President's Malaria Initiative.

The use of synthetic insecticides, particularly after an interim period of nonuse, could indeed contribute to effective malaria control and dramatically reduce childhood deaths. This was, of course, a profound benefit. Indeed, the overall impact of the second malaria eradication campaign in the period from 2002 to 2010 was estimated to have reduced overall childhood malaria deaths by 25 percent, although most of the gains could be attributed to bed net use rather than insecticide spraying.[21] The major problem with synthetic insecticides was that their effectiveness was constrained by biological laws. IRS in tropical Africa was a time-limited miracle.

[20] Donald Roberts and Richard Tren, *The Excellent Powder: DDT's Political and Scientific History* (Indianapolis: Dog Ear Publishing, 2010).
[21] Thomas P. Eisele, David A. Larsen, Neff Walker, Richard E. Cibulskis, Joshua O. Yukich, Charlotte M. Zikusooka, and Richard W. Steketee, "Estimates of Child Deaths Prevented from Malaria Prevention Scale-up in Africa 2001–2010, *Malaria Journal*, vol. 11 (2012), no. 93. Available online: http://www.malariajournal.com/content/11/1/93/

MEDICINES, OLD AND NEW

In the early twenty-first century, the second global malaria eradication campaign, like the first, accorded a significant role to chemical therapy. Vector control could significantly reduce malarial infections to very low numbers, but bed nets, IRS, environmental engineering, and larviciding could not reach the goal of zero malaria transmission.

In the second campaign, some of the older medicines still served. Medical workers no longer prescribed chloroquine, and public health authorities no longer recommended its use, yet substantial quantities of the venerable drug continued to circulate. Its reputation was well established, and many sufferers continued to take the drug even when it had lower efficacy. For some adults, chloroquine functioned in the same manner as the better indigenous therapies: it reduced the parasite load and made the sick feel better, even if it did not clear the infection. The venerable pyrimethamine, in combination with sulfadoxine, also served well as an antimalarial until widespread resistance emerged in the 1990s, but it too continued to be sought out for use.[22]

Chloroquine began to appear in a new light as researchers discovered new evolutionary dynamics. In Malawi, where chloroquine use had been largely phased out in the late 1990s, the parasites began to lose their resistance to the drug in the absence of selection pressure. The possibility of a new chloroquine era glittered. Research suggested that much larger doses of chloroquine might act via other pathways on the malaria parasite without producing toxic reactions in the sick person.[23]

By far the most important chemotherapeutic breakthrough, however, was in the discovery of the antimalarial properties of *Artemisia annua*, a common plant whose virtues had been recorded in the ancient Chinese materia medica.[24] The antimalarial properties of the plant were explored during the era of the Cultural Revolution (1966–1976) in China. Knowledge of this "new" antimalarial outside of China was slow to be developed. The first Western medical contacts after the Cultural Revolution took place in

---

[22] Foreign travelers to Africa were frequently prescribed antimalarial drugs other than chloroquine and SP. One of these drugs – mefloquine (trade name: Lariam) – was discovered to produce dangerous psychological side effects.

[23] J. H. Ch'ng, L. Renia, F. Nosten, and K. S. W. Tan, "Can We Teach an Old Drug New Tricks?," *Trends in Parasitology*, vol. 28, no. 6 (2012), 220–224.

[24] The first written commentary appeared in the third century CE. On the rediscovery of the antimalarial properties of *Artemisia annua*, see Elisabeth Hsu, "Reflections on the 'Discovery' of the Antimalarial Qinghao," *British Journal of Clinical Pharmacology*, vol. 61, no. 6 (2006), 666–670.

1980, and the World Health Organization (WHO) did not begin investigations into drugs based on the compounds in *Artemisia annua* until the early 1990s; it began to promote their use only in 2004.[25] Great hopes accompanied the introduction of artemisinin-based drugs. The seemingly sudden arrival of a new, front-line antimalarial – one that could be combined with some of the older drugs to slow down the emergence of resistance – opened new prospects for saving lives and reducing suffering. Early in the twenty-first century, the new chemical therapies, however, were far more expensive than chloroquine had been during the first eradication campaign.

The new antimalarial drugs on the markets were also less reliable than other pharmaceuticals at any point in the long history of malaria control. As pharmaceutical companies in tropical Africa, India, China, Brazil, and elsewhere began to produce them, the prices that they could command were high enough to encourage counterfeit and fraud. Poorly manufactured or fully ersatz drugs flowed into market stalls across Africa. When the drugs contained no active antimalarial ingredients, the sufferers received no benefits and lost confidence in the medicines. When the drugs were adulterated and contained lower than therapeutic doses, they promoted the emergence and spread of parasite resistance. The quantities of substandard drugs on the African markets were considerable; researchers suggested that as much as 50 percent of all drugs in some regions of Africa were counterfeit.[26]

The new artemisinin-based drugs were based on natural alkaloids that had to be extracted directly from the *Artemisia annua* plant. Large-scale plantations had to be laid out to produce the wonder alkaloids, in a reprise of the efforts to grow cinchona trees for their alkaloids on plantations in tropical Africa in the 1930s and 1940s, in the era before chloroquine. Fortunately, *Artemisia annua* was not nearly as difficult to grow as the cinchona tree, and, by the middle of the first decade of the twenty-first century, highland plantations in Kenya, Uganda, and Tanzania were well on the way to meeting the growing demand.[27]

Combined with other antimalarial compounds, these artemisinin combination therapies (ACTs) became front-line drugs in the battle to save

[25] On the movement of artemisinin from China to the "global stage," see Dana G. Dalrymple, *Artemisia annua, Artemisinin, ACTs, and Malaria Control in Africa: Tradition, Science, and Public Policy* (Washington, DC: Politics and Prose Bookstore, 2012), 17–23.

[26] R. Cockburn, P. N. Newton, E. K. Agyarko, D. Akunyili, and N. J. White, "The Global Threat of Counterfeit Drugs: Why Industry and Governments Must Communicate the Dangers," *PLOS Medicine*, vol. 2, no. 4 (2005), 302–308.

[27] Dalrymple, *Artemisia annua, Artemisinin, ACTs, and Malaria Control in Africa.*

lives. The high cost of the drugs, however, made it difficult for many sufferers to afford the recommended course of treatment. Many bought their medications from local shopkeepers a few pills at a time, and, when the symptoms receded, stopped taking them. This pattern of use produced in vivo conditions in which the parasites were exposed to lower-than-optimal doses of the ACTs and thereby inadvertently encouraged the emergence of resistance.

As the use of ACTs began to save lives in Africa, storm clouds appeared almost immediately on the eastern horizon. Researchers documented resistance to artemisinin in Cambodia and understood that it was only a matter of time before it spread to tropical Africa.[28]

The power of the antimalarial drugs, however, was still formidable and would remain so for a number of years, and the drugs were put to therapeutic purposes beyond the strictly curative. On a trial-and-error basis, physicians developed a range of preventative regimens that could limit the damage from severe falciparum infections when the body's immune system was immature or otherwise unable to do so.

The empirical roots of what came to be known as *intermittent preventive therapy* (IPT) reached back into the first half of the twentieth century, when physicians in the Belgian colonies had discovered that giving intermittent doses of quinine to young children, even when they were not presenting with malarial symptoms, produced large improvements in morbidity and mortality. This knowledge does not seem to have diffused beyond the Belgian colonies, and it was apparently lost during the first eradication era and the chaotic transition to political independence.

A half century later, in the 1980s, the Americans discovered that women who were pregnant for the first time were particularly at risk for severe malaria, even if their immune responses to malarial infections had been robust before pregnancy. On a trial-and-error basis, the women were given antimalarial drugs, and this therapy (IPTp) prevented a great deal of severe illness and saved the lives of mothers and their unborn children.

---

[28] Arjen M. Dondorp, Shunmay Yeung, Lisa White, Chea Nguon, Nicholas P. J. Day, Duong Socheat, and Lorenz von Seidlein, "Artemisinin Resistance: Current Status and Scenarios for Containment," *Nature Reviews Microbiology*, vol. 8, no. 4 (2010), 272–280. The earlier resistance to chloroquine had emerged in the same Southeast Asian subregion in the context of a medicated salt project. J. Verdrager, "Epidemiology of Emergence and Spread of Drug-Resistant Falciparum Malaria in Southeast Asia," *Southeast Asian Journal of Tropical Medicine and Public Health*, vol. 17, no. 1 (1986), 111–118.

Later, physicians extended the practice of IPT to infants (IPTi) and young children (IPTc). The results were extremely encouraging. No one knew exactly how the therapy worked: the IPT regimens did not stave off all malarial infections or prevent all deaths and serious complications, but it was a major intervention. For those who had access to primary care, the IPT regimens saved more lives than did the insecticide-treated bed nets. It was a powerful argument for the extension of PHC. Yet, in a politicized global health environment in which global donors were skeptical of building health systems and preferred to concentrate on vertical programs, the case for the extension of PHC was rarely advanced.

The problem of emerging drug resistance was grave. The economic incentives ran counter to public health need. An aggressive program of new drug development would be very expensive, and its potential market would be poor people who got malaria and could barely pay for their medications. In 1999, a private–public partnership known as Medicines for Malaria Venture was launched in an effort to serve as a clearinghouse for potentially useful drug candidates, and, in 2012, a new synthetic ozonide passed the first trials. This compound was among the most promising advances in malaria treatment and control because, if it could be brought to market later in the decade, the ozonide would likely provide front-line treatment after the anticipated spread of artemisinin resistance.[29] It was a flicker of light at the end of a long tunnel.

MALARIA AND HIV

The juggernaut of burgeoning HIV, tubercular, and malarial infections in the 1990s had called forth a new era of global health interventions in the form of separate vertical programs for the three diseases. It was clear, however, that HIV and tubercular infections were integrally dynamic and that the explosion in the number of TB cases in tropical Africa was in large measure a function of the spread of HIV. The HIV infections degraded the immune system and allowed for latent TB infections to become active, and those with active infections could spread TB to others.

---

[29] Jörg Möhrle, Stephan Duparc, Christoph Siethoff, Paul L. M. van Giersbergen, J. Carl Craft, Sarah Arbe-Barnes, Susan A. Charman, Maria Gutierrez, Sergio Wittlin, and Jonathan L. Vennerstrom, "First-in-Man Safety and Pharmacokinetics of Synthetic Ozonide OZ439 Demonstrates an Improved Exposure Profile Relative to Other Peroxide Antimalarials," *British Journal of Clinical Pharmacology*, vol. 75, no. 2 (2013), 535–548.

The epidemiological relationship between HIV and malaria, however, was not scientifically established until 2005. This was largely a result of the compartmentalization engendered by vertical programs. In retrospect, it seemed obvious that HIV infections would disable the immune system and make it more difficult to suppress the malaria parasites, that the higher parasite loads would mean more severe disease among those with presenting symptoms, and that higher parasite loads, in turn, might make those infected with both HIV and malaria able to transmit more gametocytes to the hungry anophelines. HIV might thereby be indicted as a multiplier of malarial infections. There was, however, a silver lining to this cloud, even if badly tarnished: the artemisinin-based therapies that targeted the malaria parasites powerfully reduced the viral HIV load of malaria sufferers who were HIV positive.[30]

THE VACCINE TRIALS

The Bill and Melinda Gates Foundation's commitment to malaria eradication was, within a few years, recast as "malaria elimination," a semantic turn that deflected comparisons with the first unsuccessful global malaria eradication program and a belated recognition that eradication would not be achieved in the foreseeable future. The Gates Foundation's research program focused on the search for a vaccine. The hope, as ever, was that an effective vaccine might solve the malaria problem once and for all. To the layperson, the approach seemed commonsensical because an array of vaccines had proved highly effective against many of the ancient scourges of humanity. In the case of smallpox, the vaccine had eradicated the disease. And other vaccines – such as that for polio – had greatly reduced the number of cases, to the point at which the prospects for eventual eradication appeared to be good. Other vaccines didn't promise eradication in the near term, but those for measles, rubella, diphtheria, pertussis, rotavirus, and others had largely staunched these diseases among vaccinated populations.

The successful vaccines worked by introducing antigens that stimulated the immune system's antibodies against pathogenic bacteria and viruses. There were, however, no vaccines for human beings that worked against

[30] A. Lubbe, I. Seibert, T. Klimkait, and F. van der Kooy, "Ethnopharmacology in Overdrive: The Remarkable Anti-HIV Activity of *Artemisia annua*," *Journal of Ethnopharmacology*, vol. 141, no. 3 (2012), 854–859.

any of the pathogenic parasites.[31] The one-celled *Plasmodium falciparum* organism was amazingly complex. It had 5,300 genes, and half of them had neither a known function nor a counterpart in any other organism. Moreover, each of the four different life stages of the falciparum parasite had a different array of genes that governed the synthesis of antigens.[32]

The search for an effective and safe malaria vaccine had progressed in fits and starts for several generations, and, by the early twenty-first century, there were several different approaches.[33] The most clinically advanced vaccine candidacy was that of RTS,S, in development since 1987. In 2011, RTS,S went through the first stage of phase III trials. It offered protection against severe malaria to about half of those aged 5–17 months who received the vaccine, and less protection for a younger group aged 6–12 weeks. In 2012, another phase III trial showed only modest efficacy against clinical malaria in the 6- to 12-week-old group.[34] The RTS,S vaccine was far from perfect. It provided only partial protection, and it had to be administered in a series of three shots – a requirement that might prove to be an insurmountable obstacle in much of tropical Africa, where populations were poorly served by even rudimentary medical services. Yet, RTS,S held promise as an additional measure that might be deployed to reduce the incidence of severe malaria and to reduce malaria deaths. For its advocates, the RTS,S vaccine was a glass half full.

There were two fundamentally different approaches to vaccine making. The RTS,S vaccine candidate targeted those stages in the parasite life cycle before its invasion of red blood cells. The goal was to prevent the progression of infectious stages that led to disease. The gold standard was 100 percent protection. In a sense, it was an approach that harkened back to the core issue of the colonial period: how to keep European nonimmunes safe in tropical African environments. It had immediate military significance. If the vaccine could be used to protect nonimmune combat

[31] For an overview of the status of and prospects for antiparasitic vaccines for use in animals, see J. Vercruysse, T. P. M. Schetters, D. P. Knox, P. Willadsen, and E. Claerebout, "Control of Parasitic Disease Using Vaccines: An Answer to Drug Resistance?," *Revue scientifique et technique de l'Office International des Epizooties*, vol. 26, no. 1 (2007), 105–115.

[32] Sherman, *Elusive Malaria Vaccine*, 341.

[33] The outstanding history of the search for a malaria vaccine is Sherman's *The Elusive Malaria Vaccine*.

[34] The RTS,S Clinical Trials Partnership, "First Results of Phase 3 Trial of RTS,S/AS01 Malaria Vaccine in African Children," *New England Journal of Medicine*, vol. 365 (2011), 1863–75; The RTS,S Clinical Trials Partnership, "A Phase 3 Trial of RTS,S/AS01 Malaria Vaccine in African Children," *New England Journal of Medicine*, vol. 367 (2012), 2284–2295.

troops, it would allow for their deployment in malarial areas without risk of infection. It could reduce, for example, the health risks of operations against Islamist groups in tropical Africa.

A radically different approach looked at the problem of malaria from the perspective of the partially immune. From this point of view, the core problem was not the prevention of infection. It was how to reduce the severity of infection and thereby allow for the development of a robust natural immunological response. Its approach was to try to boost the immune system and thereby prevent the consequences of severe infection. This was of little interest to the US military because it would not prevent malaria.[35]

NEW VULNERABILITIES

As the control programs advanced in many states across tropical Africa (and faltered in the war zones), and as new advances were registered in the North Atlantic laboratories, distressing findings from the malaria front lines began to cast the entire control strategy in a new light.

It had long been known that highly successful malaria control efforts would compromise the immunological responses of populations that were no longer challenged by malarial infections. This was a relatively minor problem if the control efforts could be sustained over time and those with compromised immunological defenses who moved into areas of transmission in theory could be provided treatment. According to the grand schemes of malaria eradication in the 1950s and 1960s and malaria "elimination" in the 2000s and 2010s, malaria control would increase in effectiveness over time. The visions were of a progressive reduction in malaria transmission toward the ultimate achievement of zero transmission. The vision was an epidemiological one, grounded in a set of interactions linking parasites, vectors, and control interventions that paid scant attention to the unpredictable immune responses of those who sustained many fewer infections. It was at once scientifically rigorous and blinkered.

In Senegal, French and Senegalese scientists had long tracked the morbidity and mortality of populations that had benefited from malaria control efforts. One of the senior malariologists, Jean-François Trape, had signaled the tragedy that ensued from the spread of chloroquine-resistant

---

[35] The leading proponent of this approach was Louis J. Miller of the National Institute for Allergy and Infectious Disease (NIAID).

strains of falciparum.[36] As the malaria control efforts in the early twenty-first century spread throughout Senegal, significantly reducing deaths and severe sickness, scientific monitoring efforts continued. In the village of Dielmo, the people had accepted bed net use and achieved a high rate of coverage that allowed them to enjoy community-level benefits that extended to those who did not use the nets. Moreover, the villagers had access to artemisinin-based combination therapies for those who came down with clinical attacks of malaria. Transmission rates were low, and the general health of the population improved. The levels of individual acquired immunity began to degrade.

Then, pyrethroid resistance began to develop. The nets were no longer as epidemiologically effective. They still worked by using humans as bait to cause the mosquitoes to pick up the insecticides, but some of the mosquitoes did not die before the parasites developed within them and those mosquitoes took another blood meal. Transmission began to rise, although not to levels known before the bed net intervention. The researchers suspected that those who once had robust immunities had become more susceptible to severe malaria. The findings were treated as novel, although they were consonant with earlier experiences with lapsed malaria control, dating back to the earliest documented experiences in Freetown, Sierra Leone, in the aftermath of the Second World War. The findings sent frissons of fear and concern throughout the malaria control community. Their data suggested that the road to elimination would be bumpy indeed and that the distribution of the burden of disease might be shifted to different age cohorts.[37]

In the lowlands of Madagascar, those villagers who had adopted the insecticide-treated bed nets, like the villagers in Dielmo, began to experience a marked decrease in morbidity and mortality. As in Senegal, the efficacy of the insecticide-treated bed nets had been bolstered by access to artemisinin-based combination therapies. The nets alone had worked wonders. But the effective lifespan of the nets – and the insecticides applied

---

[36] Jean-François Trape, "The Public Health Impact of Chloroquine Resistance in Africa," 12–17.

[37] J. -F. Trape, A. Tall, N. Diagne, O. Ndiath, A. B. Ly, J. Faye, F. Dieye-Ba, C. Roucher, C. Bouganali, A. Badiane, F. Diene Sarr, C. Mazenot, A. Touré-Baldé, D. Raoult, P. Druilhe, O. Mercereau-Puijalon, C. Rogier, and C. Sokhna, "Malaria Morbidity and Pyrethroid Resistance after the Introduction of Insecticide-treated Bed Nets Artemisinin-based Combination Therapies: A Longitudinal Study," *Lancet Infectious Diseases*, vol. 11, no. 12 (2011), 925–932. See also the responses to this article in Sylla Thiam, Rumishael Shoo, and Jane Carter, "Are Insecticide Treated Bednets Failing?," *Lancet Infectious Diseases*, vol. 12, no. 7 (2012), 512–514.

to them – had proved shorter than predicted, and the interventionists had not laid down plans to replace the nets. During the short years of effective protection, the acquired immunities of the Madagascan villagers degraded. Local epidemiological variables helped to determine these new vulnerabilities. Heavier than normal rains increased the density of the vector mosquitoes. Shortages in the available supplies of artemisinin meant that many cases of severe malaria could not be effectively treated. In 2012, as the combination of malaria control measures weakened, outbreaks of epidemic malaria flared.

These vulnerabilities were decidedly not signs of any kind of general breakdown of malaria control. They were, in a sense, symptoms of success. The overall advances in bed net coverage meant that there were progressive gains in lives saved and sickness prevented. Yet, the evidence from Senegal and Madagascar underscored the fact that the typical programs of malaria control would have difficulties in consolidating their gains. Ongoing malaria control and the ability to intervene to reverse serious adverse events depended on access to medications, as well as on bed nets.

FINANCIAL VULNERABILITIES

The achievements of the malaria elimination program depended on financial resources that flowed into tropical Africa. The money spigot had gurgled in the early years of the decade and opened up to a full stream by 2007–2008, when bed nets began to flood across the continent. Large sums flowed to research centers where vaccines, transgenic mosquitoes, and new bacterial and fungal infections to prevent the development of the parasite within the anophelines were under design.

But in 2008, a global financial crisis took deep root, and although frantic government policy-makers managed to forestall a general economic paralysis, economic growth slowed in many regions of the world, producing multiple centers of economic malaise. The European economies were beset by an intransigent economic crisis that had its roots in the absence of an integrated European Union (EU) monetary system. The net result was that, facing the prospect of a deepening economic and political crisis in Europe, EU countries reduced their commitments to the Global Fund. There was less money to go around, and the malaria projects were unable to expand their programs. The open question was for just how long the developed countries would be willing to commit monies for malaria control. The rhetoric of "elimination," like the earlier rhetoric of eradication, might prove to be an elixir with a short shelf life.

POLITICAL VULNERABILITIES

Beyond the issue of finance, many interventionists came to appreciate more fully that the political commitment of African governments was a sine qua non of ongoing control. The African scientific community was fully on board, but its political influence varied greatly from one state to the next. In the short and medium term, the political commitment of African states could be secured through bilateral grants to fund control programs, training opportunities, and staff salaries. But health and development projects typically operated on multiyear cycles. They were not open-ended. Government functionaries in many African states siphoned off monies, and, as the extent of corruption within the Global Fund projects began to come to light, international support weakened.

Another critical dimension of malaria politics was local. Malaria control specialists learned that buy-in from local African communities was key. Communities had to understand the interventions and value them. This would entail a project of medical education that was deeply cross-cultural and would depend upon the efforts of individuals who knew regional languages and idioms and who were versed in the translation of concepts of disease, prevention, and cure. This was a kind of capacity building that was far beyond the simple distribution of insecticide treated bed nets.

A wildcard variable was the potential for political instability. Many of the African states born during the independence struggles of the mid and late twentieth centuries had been racked with political conflicts in the twenty-first century. Some had descended into warlordism. The penchant of some members of the global health community – and the malaria control community – to plan interventions without a realistic consideration of the prospects for political instability meant that there were additional elements of uncertainty that might translate into failure. In conflict zones, efforts at malaria control were practically futile.

In states with stable politics, by contrast, outcomes were strongly positive. In Senegal, for example, remarkable gains had been made in extending bed net coverage, IPTp, and artemisinin-based therapies. The number of malaria cases dropped considerably. Similar gains were realized in other African states, including Zambia and Kenya.[38] The African political map

---

[38] Roll Back Malaria, "Focus on Senegal." This report was one in the Progress Impact Series. Available online: http://www.rollbackmalaria.org/ProgressImpactSeries/report4.html

was diverse, and a common program of malaria control strategies would produce highly divergent health outcomes and patterns of vulnerabilities.

WITHOUT AN ENDGAME

The second great malaria intervention was launched without an endgame. It was known that the existing control measures could be powerfully effective. They could greatly reduce transmission, but no matter the combinations of interventions or intensities with which they were deployed, they would not be capable of completely interrupting transmission. One hope was that with enough research monies flowing into laboratories a technological solution would be found.[39]

In some sense, the dangers of embarking on a large-scale program to control malaria were real enough. The repeated injunctions in the 1980s to privatize health care in Africa had resulted in the weakening of many rural health care facilities.[40] Absent an ongoing flow of resources to African malaria control, much of the effort might collapse. A repeat of the severe malaria epidemics that followed the first great malaria intervention was well within the realm of possibility.

The spread of resistance to the front-line insecticides used on bed nets was well advanced. The resistance to artemisinin had emerged in Southeast Asia, and it was generally understood that it was only a matter of time before it made its way to Africa and began to spread throughout the continent, as had chloroquine resistance during the first great malaria intervention.

Yet another seed of danger lay in the dynamics of the early successes of the malaria control programs. As ever, the most impressive gains were to be had in the first years of control, when infections could be driven to low levels. Thereafter lay a future of open-ended control with substantial recurrent costs and new investments in surveillance. In the second malaria eradication program, the surveillance problem was reconfigured by the widespread use of rapid diagnostic tests. This promised to reduce the expense of one important aspect of long-term control. But the other interventions – bed nets, insecticides, and antimalarial drugs – would remain expensive and their availability uncertain. In the past, the ability

---

[39] Some found this vision inspirational. See, for example, William H. Shore, *The Imaginations of Unreasonable Men: Inspiration, Vision, and Purpose in the Quest to End Malaria* (New York: Public Affairs, 2010).

[40] Ellen E. Foley, *Your Pocket Is What Cures You: The Politics of Health in Senegal* (New Brunswick, NJ: Rutgers University Press, 2010).

to carry out malaria control had faced stiff competition for scarce resources. When other illnesses caused more immediate suffering and death, it had proved near impossible to make the case for ongoing malaria control.

LOOKING AHEAD

The risks of waning interest in African malaria were palpable. In part to bolster support for malaria elimination, the Roll Back Malaria program touted a near-term goal of zero preventable malaria deaths by 2015. Taken at face value, this was obviously unachievable, given that, by any count, there were many hundreds of thousands of deaths occurring every year in tropical Africa.[41]

Some within the Roll Back Malaria program argued that there was no harm in promoting an unrealistic goal, with the view that this would spur donors to continue their financial contributions. From an historical vantage point, however, this was grounds for serious concern. The first malaria eradication program had overpromised, and its inability to reach its lofty goal had been interpreted as a humiliating defeat. This had dampened interest in malaria control for more than a generation, even though, by other measures, the first global malaria eradication program had been a large success. It had dramatically reduced malarial sickness and death by an order of magnitude outside of tropical Africa.

During the current malaria eradication campaign, the most realistic and best hope is that similarly significant gains might be achieved and sustained in tropical Africa, even though the tools that are currently available are not sufficient to fully interrupt malaria transmission. The best that can be achieved in the medium term is a system of ongoing malaria control that will reduce malaria transmission to low levels and an upgraded system of PHC that will make intermittent preventive therapy available to pregnant women, infants, and children and medical treatment available to those who contract severe infections.

Malaria control initiatives will have to be tailored to African realities. Ongoing malaria control will have to be carried out by national malaria services, and this will require a major effort to train personnel and fund

---

[41] The methodologies to estimate malaria deaths had undergone a number of major revisions. The rapid diagnostic tests suggested that malaria was quantitatively a smaller problem than had been previously thought. Then new quantitative studies, funded by the Gates Foundation, made the case that the number of malaria deaths per year was far higher than had been previously imagined. See Murray et al., "Global Malaria Mortality between 1980 and 2010," 413–431.

these services. Such an ongoing financial commitment to national malaria services will involve the devolution of malaria control to African actors, who will need to focus their efforts on local epidemiological challenges. Even under close to ideal circumstances, the spatial distribution of effective malaria control will be uneven, and its successes will reflect in part the broader strengths of state institutional structures. Weak states will not be able to achieve ongoing malaria control. Into the foreseeable future, the most that can be hoped for is a patchwork of successes.

7

Perspectives

The contemporary campaign to control malaria in tropical Africa, based principally on the distribution of insecticide-treated bed nets and the indoor spraying of residual insecticides, has produced highly impressive results. It has substantially reduced deaths and severe illnesses. The contemporary efforts to diagnose malarial infections accurately and to treat infected individuals with artemisinin-based combination therapies (ACTs) have saved lives and reduced the medical sequelae from severe infections. Yet in the midst of these successes, there have been some disturbing and predictable trends. The use of insecticides has selected for resistance in the vector mosquitoes, and insecticides in a growing number of settings have become less effective in killing the mosquitoes. Resistance to artemisinin is spreading in Southeast Asia, and most experts consider it only a matter of time before artemisinin resistance reaches tropical Africa.

Thus, in some important respects, the current campaign is repeating some of the core experiences of the first aborted attempt at malaria eradication in tropical Africa. There are remarkable continuities. Indeed, many of the focused attempts at full control or elimination have taken place in the same zones as the mid-twentieth century efforts. A frequently cited example is the island of Zanzibar, which participated in an eradication program in the 1960s, undertook a second effort at control in the 1980s, and is now undergoing its third campaign. From this perspective, malaria control can appear to be a Sisyphean endeavor.

The biological controls that can be exercised over malaria transmission have real limitations. No combination of new malaria control or treatment tools in the pipeline can assure the full and sustainable interruption of transmission, and thus it seems certain that the goal of malaria eradication (or "elimination" in contemporary parlance) will remain out of reach in the short and medium term.

Yet, to consider the current campaign a simple replay of the first eradication campaign would be to ignore the vast changes that have taken place over the past fifty years. Tropical Africa in the early twenty-first century is far more technologically integrated by virtue of the communications revolution based on cell phones and personal computers. In some areas, this integration gives health care providers an ability to diagnose and treat the symptomatic more quickly. There is more buy-in among some African governments to the project of malaria control and elimination than in the past, and some African governments have made moderate financial commitments to it. The very face of malaria control – that is, the cadres of African scientists, physicians, nurses, and public health workers – has changed. In some important respects, malaria eradication is no longer solely a project of the Global North.

In some important respects, malaria control in tropical Africa has become more culturally diverse. Indeed, even as ACTs become accepted as the front-line drug to treat malarial infections, a burgeoning African pharmaceutical industry has developed to market African treatments that have not been vetted by the biomedical community. China has a growing presence in tropical Africa that extends far beyond the well-appreciated programs of infrastructure development. Africans are expressing growing interest in the Chinese drugs that are available in many African cities. These developments lie outside the focus of the biomedical community and have been little investigated.

The Global North, however, is still the primary funder of the project of malaria control or elimination, and this represents a marked continuity with the aborted mid-twentieth century eradication campaign. In the years after the 2008 global financial crisis, the resources available for malaria control were cut back and now are insufficient to realize the goals of the malaria control community. This is a repeat of what occurred in the mid-twentieth century. It seems unlikely, given the tepid rate of economic growth in the United States and the ongoing economic crisis in Europe, that more governmental financial support will become available for malaria control in tropical Africa.

The same may not be true in the philanthropic sector. In 2013, the Bill and Melinda Gates Foundation moved toward the implementation of a new paradigm of malaria eradication – one focused on the development of new medicines for individual, radical cures to be used in combination with a drug to kill malaria gametocytes, with the hope of clearing the parasitic infections of both symptomatic and asymptomatic individuals. The program is anticipated to incur heavy initial costs. The hope is that, in areas in which malarial infections have been driven to low numbers by IRS and bed nets, these drug interventions can deliver the coup de grâce.

Early in the twentieth century, European-trained physicians recognized a principal epidemiological difference between the response to malaria of nonimmune Europeans and partially immune Africans. The nature, role, and duration of the immunological response to infection known generically as acquired immunity was deemed to be of critical importance in shaping malaria interventions. For Europeans who were in power during the colonial period, assumptions about the significance of acquired immunity helped to determine whether Africans should receive chemical therapies and, if so, the dosage regimens that were appropriate. Medical perceptions of the different experiences of the nonimmune European and the partially immune African shaped European-led efforts to control malaria in the era before the Second World War.

The issue of acquired immunity was central to European ways of thinking about African malaria in the interwar period, and it reemerged in the immediate aftermath of the Second World War, when a highly successful malaria control effort in Freetown, Sierra Leone, lapsed and resurgent malaria afflicted older age cohorts who had lost their acquired immunities to malaria during the period of successful interventions. It was central to the debates over whether to attempt the eradication of malaria in rural Africa during the build-up to the World Health Organization (WHO)'s global Malaria Eradication Program. It reemerged again, following the closure of the WHO malaria eradication pilot projects, when resurgent malaria struck some of the populations that had been protected from infection during the life of the pilot projects. It looms as an issue in the context of the contemporary campaigns to control or eliminate malaria, as malaria interventions in some areas have become less effective.

When malaria programs have lapsed after a number of years of successful control, "rebound" epidemic malaria has afflicted formerly protected communities, and the health consequences of these epidemics have gone largely unmeasured. In part, this may be because the metaphor of the "rebound" suggests that the disease has "bounced back" to or below its preintervention levels. The logic of the metaphor implies that, because the loss of control results in the re-establishment of infection at or below a preexisting equilibrium, African communities could be no worse off than they would have been otherwise.

Yet evidence from as early as the 1940s indicates that lapsed malaria control has resulted in the loss of acquired immunities among populations and the emergence of new vulnerabilities. When malaria transmission has been re-established, even at far lower levels than previously, some of the burden of disease is shifted to those in older age cohorts who had previously enjoyed greater protection by virtue of their acquired immunities. For older individuals and those who suffer from human immunodeficiency virus (HIV) infection or other infections that compromise the immune response, the re-establishment of malaria transmission will cause an increase in serious illness and death. Whether this is true of younger age cohorts is not known.

This question, with its medical and ethical dimensions, has not received much study. In part, this may be because the gains in lives saved in the "protected" populations appear to be far greater than any damage caused by lapses in control. When the measure of benefit is the number of lives saved, the cost–benefit ratio is powerfully favorable to malaria control, even with lapses. This utilitarian approach expresses a philosophical view that all human life has the same value, regardless of age. This perspective has taken root in societies in which infectious disease has been largely controlled and in environments in which sustenance is not principally gained by laboring in agricultural fields. In rural Africa, as in virtually all societies before the "demographic transition," the loss of a productive adult to malaria is not comparable to the loss of an infant.

The logic of the expansion of highly effective yet potentially unsustainable public health measures has held the day because malaria control has been represented as an unimpeachable good. Yet, when the phenomenon of resurgent malaria is anticipated to be a likely outcome of lapsed control or eradication efforts and there is no ironclad commitment to funding ongoing national malaria services, the moral dimensions of malaria interventions are no longer simple and straightforward. It is indisputably noble to save the life of a child. The moral calculus becomes more complex if resurgent malaria takes the life of a mother.

The contemporary malaria control and eradication programs are currently struggling to manage the heightened extent of mosquito and parasite resistance, and it is likely that some of the programs, particularly those in African states with weak institutions, will prove unsustainable. The prospects for a repeat of the epidemiological consequences of past interventions constitute a significant public health risk for contemporary African populations.

In the past, when commitments to malaria control have waned, the interventionists have enjoyed a kind of immunity from moral censure. There is no opprobrium that attaches to doing one's best and failing. With a fuller understanding of the historical record of control-and-lapse in tropical Africa, the contemporary malaria control and eradication community of donors and practitioners has an obligation to design programs that will prevent resurgent malaria. This will likely mean the development of more robust systems of public health and PHC, and this will likely only be possible in moderately or highly successful states.

Bibliography

Archives Consulted

Institut de Médicine Tropicale du Service de Santé des Armées (IMTSSA), Archives de l'Ecole du Pharo, Marseille.
London School of Hygiene and Tropical Medicine (LSHTM), Ross Archives, London.
National Archives of the United Kingdom (NAUK), Kew, Surrey.
Rhodes House Library, Oxford.
Wellcome Library, Contemporary Medical Archives Center, London.
Wellcome Unit for the History of Medicine, Malaria Room, Oxford.
World Health Organization (WHO), Parasitological Archives, Geneva.

US Government Reports

American Public Health Association. "Workshop Report. Malaria Control in PHC in Africa. Washington, DC, June 28–July 2, 1982." Available online: http://pdf.usaid.gov/pdf_docs/PNAAY965.pdf
American Public Health Association. *Manual on Malaria Control in Primary Health Care in Africa* (Washington, DC: Bureau for Africa, USAID, 1982).
Graham, B. J. "Malaria Eradication/Control Problems in Sub-Saharan Africa: Previous Programs and Factors Which Influence Successful Programs." Office of Health, Development Support Bureau, Agency for International Development, Department of State. August 1979.
USAID, Office of Health. "Report of Consultants–African Malaria [1975]." PN-AAN–885. Available online: http://pdf.usaid.gov/pdf_docs/PNAAN885.pdf
USAID, Mission to Zaire. "Draft. Review of Malaria Control Programs in Developing Countries: Zaire, Africa Country Summary," 4. PD-ABA–487 (November 1981). Available online: http://pdf.usaid.gov/pdf_docs/PDABA487.pdf
US Department of Health, Education, and Welfare. *Annual Report. Fiscal Year 1970. Malaria Program, Center for Disease Control* (Atlanta: CDC, 1970).
US Department of Health and Human Services, Public Health Service, Centers for Disease Control, International Health Program Office. *Addressing the Challenges of Malaria Control in Africa* (Washington, DC: USAID, Africa Regional Project (698–0421), n. d. [c. 1994]).

US Department of Health and Human Services, Public Health Service, Centers for Disease Control, International Health Program Office. *Controlling Malaria in Africa: Progress and Priorities* (Washington, DC: USAID, Africa Regional Project (698–0421), n. d. [c. 1994]).

US Department of Health and Human Services, Public Health Service, Centers for Disease Control, International Health Program Office. *Malaria Prevention in Pregnancy: The Mangochi Malaria Research Project* (Washington, DC: USAID, Africa Regional Project (698–0421), n.d., [c. 1993]).

World Health Organization Documents

WHO Regional Office for Africa. *Afro Malaria Eradication Yearbook No. 1* (Geneva: WHO, 1959).

WHO Regional Office for Africa. *Afro Malaria Yearbook No. 2* (Geneva: WHO, 1960).

WHO Regional Office for Africa. *Malaria Control in Africa: A Framework for the Implementation of the Regional Malaria Control Strategy, 1996–2001* (Brazzaville: WHO, Regional Office for Africa, 1996).

Websites and Hyperlinks

Centers for Disease Control. http://www.cdc.gov/MALARIA

President's Malaria Initiative. http://www.fightingmalaria.gov

Roll Back Malaria. http://www.rollbackmalaria.org. The Roll Back Malaria website provides up-to-date information on the current campaign.

World Health Organization, Malaria Publications. This link to the document WHO/MAL/2012.1119 contains hyperlinks to the entire collection of the WHO/MAL series of OFFSET documents covering the period from 1947 to 2000: http://www.who.int/malaria/publications/atoz/whomal_2012.1119.pdf

Articles and Books

Abudho, R. A., and R. A. Abudho. "The Growth of Africa's Urban Population," in James D. Tarver (ed.), *Urbanization in Africa: A Handbook* (Westport, CT: Greenwood Press, 1994), 49–64.

Achtman, A. H., P. C. Bull, R. Stephens, and J. Langhorne. "Longevity of Immune Response and Memory to Blood-Stage Malaria Infection," *Current Topics in Microbiology and Immunology*, vol. 297 (2005), 71–102.

Aikins, M. K., H. Pickering, P. L. Alonso, U. D'Alessandro, S. W. Lindsay, J. Todd, and B. M. Greenwood. "A Malaria Control Trial Using Insecticide-Treated Bed Nets and Targeted Chemoprophylaxis in a Rural Area of The Gambia, West Africa. 4. Perceptions of the Causes of Malaria and of Its Treatment and Prevention in the Study Area," *Transactions of the Royal Society of Tropical Medicine and Hygiene*, vol. 87 (1993), supplement 2, 25–30.

Aldighieri, R., J. Aldighieri, R. Oudot, and J.L. San Marco. "Évolution des campagnes de lutte contre le paludisme de 1897 à nos jours," *Médecine tropicale*, vol. 45, no. 1 (1985), 9–18.

Alonso P. L., S. W. Lindsay, J. R. M. Armstrong Schellenberg, K. Keita, P. Gomez, F. C. Shenton, A. G. Hill, G. Fegan, K. Cham, and B. M. Greenwood. "A Malaria Control Trial Using Insecticide-Treated Bed Nets and Targeted Chemoprophylaxis in a Rural Area of The Gambia, West Africa. 6. The Impact of Interventions on Mortality and Morbidity from Malaria," *Transactions of the Royal Society of Tropical Medicine and Hygiene*, vol. 87 (1993), supplement 2, 37–44.

Alves, W. "Preliminary Note on a Southern Rhodesian Experiment in Malaria Control," *South African Journal of Science* (May 1951), 289–292.

Alves, W., and D. M. Blair. "Malaria Control in Southern Rhodesia," *Journal of Tropical Medicine and Hygiene*, vol. 58, no. 12 (1955), 273–280.

Amat-Roze, J.- M., and G. Remy. "Paysage épidemiologique du paludisme dans l'espace ivioro-voltaique," *Médecine tropicale*, vol. 42, no. 4 (1982), 383–392.

Andreano, R. "Economic Issues in Disease Control and Eradication," *Social Science and Medicine*, vol. 17, no. 24 (1983), 2027–2032.

Andrews, J. A. "The United States Public Health Service Communicable Disease Center," *Public Health Reports*, vol. 61, no. 33 (1946), 1203–1210.

Annett, H. E., and J. E. Dutton. *Report of the Malaria Expedition to Nigeria of the Liverpool School of Tropical Medicine and Medical Parasitology.* Memoir IV (Liverpool: University Press of Liverpool, 1901).

Annett, H. E., J. E. Dutton, and J. H. Elliott. *Report of the Malaria Expedition to Nigeria of the Liverpool School of Tropical Medicine and Medical Parasitology. Part I: Malarial Fever, Etc.* Memoir III (Liverpool: University Press of Liverpool, 1901).

[Anon.]. "The Antimalaria Campaign. The Liverpool Malaria Expedition," *British Medical Journal*, vol. 2 (7 September 1901), 644.

[Anon.]. *Le paludisme dans la zone pilote de Bobo Dioulasso Haute-Volta* (ORSTOM, 1959).

[Anon.]. "Problems of Malaria Eradication in Africa," *WHO Chronicle*, vol. 17, no. 10 (1963), 368–375.

[Anon.]. "Situation épidémiologique de la lutte antipalustre à Madagascar en 1967," *Médicine d'Afrique Noire*, no. 6 (June 1967), 311–312.

Archibald, H. M. "Malaria in South-Western and North-Western Nigerian Communities," *Bulletin of the World Health Organization*, vol. 15, nos. 3–5 (1956), 695–709.

Asidi, A., R. N'Guessen, M. Akogbeto, C. Curtis, and M. Rowland. "Loss of Household Protection from Insecticide-Treated Nets against Pyrethroid-Resistant Mosquitoes, Benin," *Emerging Infectious Diseases*, vol. 18, no. 7 (2012), 1101–1106.

Austen, E. E. *Report of the Proceedings of the Expedition for the Study of the Causes of Malaria, Despatched to Sierra Leone, West Africa, under the Leadership of Major Ronald Ross (Late Indian Medical Service), by the Liverpool School of Tropical Diseases, July 29th 1899* (London: Her Majesty's Stationary Office, 1899).

Avidon. "Traitement de la malaria par la Diuratropineiodobenzométhylée," *Annales de la Société belge de médecine tropicale*, vol. 3, no. 3 (1923), 347–352.

Ayensu, E. "Plant and Bat Interactions in West Africa," *Annals of the Missouri Botanical Garden*, vol. 61, no. 3 (1974), 702–727.

Bado, J.-P. "La lutte contre le paludisme en Afrique central. Problèmes d'hier et d'aujourd'hui," *Enjeux*, no. 18, janvier-mars 2004, 10–13.

Baird, J. K. "Age-dependent Characteristics of Protection. V. Susceptibility to *Plasmodium falciparum*," *Annals of Tropical Medicine and Parasitology*, vol. 92, no. 4 (1998), 367–390.

Bang, Y. H., F. M. Mrope, and I. B. Sabuni. "Changes in Mosquito Populations Associated with Urbanization in East Africa," *East African Medical Journal*, vol. 54, no. 7 (1977), 403–410.

Barber, M. A. "Malaria Control Work in West Africa," *Southern Medical Journal*, vol. 25, no. 6 (1932), 649–651.

Barber, M. A., M. T. Olinger, and P. Putnam. "Studies on Malaria in Southern Nigeria," *Annals of Tropical Medicine and Parasitology*, vol. 25, nos. 3–4 (1931), 461–508.

Barber, M. A., J. B. Rice, and J. Y. Brown. "Malaria Studies on the Firestone Rubber Plantation in Liberia, West Africa," *American Journal of Hygiene*, vol. 15, no. 3 (1932), 601–633.

Barlow, R. "The Economic Effects of Malaria Eradication," *American Economic Review*, vol. 57, no. 2 (1967), 130–148.

Baudon, D., P. Carnevale, P. Ambroise-Thomas, and J. Roux. "La lutte antipaludique en Afrique: De l'éradication du paludisme au contrôle des paludismes," *Revue Epidémiologique et Santé Publique*, vol. 35 (1987), 401–415.

Baudon, D., P. Carnevale, J. J. Picq, and C. Gateff. "Aspects actuels de la lutte antipaludique en Afrique subsaharienne," *Médecine d'Afrique Noire*, vol. 34, no. 10 (1987), 801–807.

Baudon, D., J. Roux, P. Carnevale, and T. R. Guiguemde. "La chimiothérapie systematique des accés febriles: Une stratégie de relais dans la lutte contre le paludisme en milieu rural," *Médecine tropicale*, vol. 43, no. 4 (1983), 341–345.

Baudon, D. V. R., F. Darriet, and M. Huerre. "Impact de la construction d'un barrage avec retenue d'eau sur la transmission du paludisme," *Bullétin de la Société de pathologie exotique*, vol. 79, no. 1 (1986), 123–129.

Bayoh, M. N., D. K. Mathias, M. R. Odiere, F. M. Mutuku, L. Kamau, J. E. Gimnig, J. M. Vulule, W. A. Hawley, M. J. Hamel, and E. D. Walker. "*Anopheles gambie*: Historical Population Decline Associated with Regional Distribution of Insecticide-Treated Bed Nets in Western Nyanza Province, Kenya," *Malaria Journal*, vol. 9, no. 62 (2010). Available online: http://www.malariajournal.com/content/9/1/62

Beausoleil, E. G. "A Review of Present Antimalaria Activities in Africa," *Bulletin of the World Health Organization*, vol. 62, supplement (1984), 13–17.

Beck, A. *A History of the British Medical Administration of East Africa* (Cambridge, MA: Harvard University Press, 1970).

Beck, A. "History of Medicine and Health Services in Kenya (1900–1950)," in L. C. Vogel et al. (eds.), *Health and Disease in Kenya* (Nairobi: East African Literature Bureau, 1974), 90–106.

Beck, A. "Medicine and Society in Tanganyika, 1890–1930: A Historical Inquiry," *Transactions of the American Philosophical Society*, vol. 67, pt. 3 (1977), 5–59.

Beck, A. *Medicine, Tradition, and Development in Kenya and Tanzania, 1920–1970* (Waltham, MA: Crossroads Press, 1983).

Bellet, Dr. "État sanitaire de Dakar et du personnel de la marine pendant l'hivernage de 1906," *Archives de médecine navale*, vol. 87 (1907), 423–428.

Benasseni, R., P. Gazin, P. Carnevale, and D. Baudon. "Le paludisme urbain à Bobo-Dioulasso (Burkina Faso)," *Cahiers ORSTOM*, série Entomologie médicale et Parasitologie, vol. 25, nos. 3–4 (1987), 15–170.

Bennett, H. L. "Anti-Malarial Drainage," *Kenya and East African Medical Journal*, vol. 7, no. 7 (1930), 190–198.

Biswas, K., I. Chattopadhyay, R. K. Banerjee, and U. Bandyopadhyay. "Biological Activities and Medicinal Properties of Neem (*Azadirachta indica*)," *Current Science*, vol. 82, no. 11 (2002), 1336–1345.

Björkman, A., J. Brohult, P. O Pehrson, M. Willcox, L. Rombo, P. Hedman, E. Kollie, K. Alestig, A. Hanson, and E. Bengtsson. "Monthly Antimalarial Chemotherapy to Children in a Holoendemic Area of Liberia," *Annals of Tropical Medicine and Parasitology*, vol. 80, no. 2 (1986), 155–167.

Björkman, A., P. Hedman, J. Brohult, M. Willcox, I. Diamant, P. O. Pehrsson, L. Rombo, and E. Bengtsson. "Different Malaria Control Activities in an Area of Liberia – Effects on Malariometric Parameters," *Annals of Tropical Medicine and Parasitology*, vol. 79, no. 3 (1985), 239–246.

Blackie, W. K. *Malaria with Special Reference to the African Forms* (Cape Town: Post-Graduate Press, 1947).

Blacklock, D. B., and R. M. Gordon. "Malaria Infection as It Occurs in Late Pregnancy, Its Relationship to Labour and Early Infancy," *Annals of Tropical Medicine and Parasitology*, vol. 19, no. 3 (1925), 327–363.

Blanchy, S., A. Rakotonjanabelo, G. Ranaivoson, and E. Rajaonarivelo. "Epidémiologie du paludisme sur les hautes terres malgaches depuis 1878," *Cahiers Santé*, vol. 3 (1993), 155–161.

Bledsoe, C. H., and M. F. Goubaud. "The Reinterpretation of Western Pharmaceuticals among the Mende of Sierra Leone," *Social Science Medicine*, vol. 21, no. 3 (1985), 275–282.

Board on Science and Technology for International Development, National Research Council. *Neem: A Tree for Solving Global Problems* (Washington, DC: National Academy Press, 1992).

Borts, G. H., H. E. Klarman, and P. Newman. "Discussion," *American Economic Review*, vol. 57, no. 2 (1967), 155–157.

Boudin, C., V. Robert, J. P. Verhave, P. Carnevale, and P. Ambroise-Thomas. "*Plasmodium falciparum* and *P. malariae* Epidemiology in a West African Village," *Bulletin of the World Health Organization*, vol. 69, no. 2 (1991), 199–205.

Bourguignon, G. -C. "Notes sur le paludisme à Elisabethville," *Annales de la Société belge de médecine tropicale*, vol. 20, no. 4 (1930), 419–460.

Boyce, R., A. Evans, and H. H. Clarke. *Report on the Sanitation and Anti-Malarial Measures in Practice in Bathurst, Conakry, and Freetown* (London: University Press of Liverpool, 1905).

Brabin, B. J. "An Analysis of Malaria in Pregnancy in Africa," *Bulletin of the World Health Organization*, vol. 61, no. 6 (1983), 1005–1016.

Bradley, D. J. "Malaria: Old Infections, Changing Epidemiology," *Health Transitions Review*, vol. 2, supplementary issue (1992), 137–153.

Bradshaw, D., and I. M. Timaeus. "Levels and Trends of Adult Mortality," in D. T. Jamison, R. G. Feacham, M. W. Makgoba, E. R. Bos, F. K. Baingana, K. J. Hofman, and K. O. Rogo (eds.), *Disease and Mortality in Sub-Saharan Africa* (Washington, DC: World Bank, 2006), 31–42.

Bremen, J. G., and C. C. Campbell. "Combating Severe Malaria in African Children," *Bulletin of the World Health Organization*, vol. 66, no. 5 (1988), 611–620.

Brinkmann, U., and A. Brinkman. "Malaria and Health in Africa: The Present Situation and Epidemiological Trends," *Tropical Medicine and Parasitology*, vol. 42 (1991), 204–213.

Brögger, R. C., H. M. Mathews, J. Storey, T. S. Ashkar, S. Brögger, and L. Molineaux. "Changing Patterns in the Humoral Immune Response to Malaria before, during, and after the Application of Control Measures: A Longitudinal Study in the West African Savanna," *Bulletin of the World Health Organization*, vol. 56, no. 4 (1978), 579–600.

Brohult, J., L. Jorfeldt, L. Rombo, A. Björkman, P. O. Pehrson, V. Sirleaf, and E. Bengtsson. "The Working Capacity of Liberian Males: A Comparison between Urban and Rural Populations in Relation to Malaria," *American Journal of Tropical Medicine and Parasitology*, vol. 75, no. 5 (1981), 487–494.

Brown, C., and J. P. Stanfield. *Medicine and Health in Africa: A Bibliography with Critical Abstracts* (London: Bureau of Hygiene and Tropical Diseases [LSHTM], 1988–1991).

Brown, P. J. "Failure as Success: Multiple Meanings of Eradication in the Rockefeller Foundation Sardinia Project," *Parassitologia*, vol. 40 (1998), 117–130.

Brown, S. H. "Public Health in Lagos, 1850–1900: Perceptions, Patterns, and Perspectives," *International Journal of African Historical Studies*, vol. 25, no. 2 (1992), 337–360.

Bruce, M. C., C. A. Donnelly, M. P. Alpers, M. R. Galinski, J. W. Barnwell, D. Walliker, and K. P. Day. "Cross-Species Interactions between Malaria Parasites in Humans," *Science*, vol. 287 (4 February 2000), 845–848.

Bruce-Chwatt, L. J. "Malaria in African Infants and Children in Southern Africa," *Annals of Tropical Medicine and Parasitology*, vol. 46, no. 2 (1952), 173–200.

Bruce-Chwatt, L. J. "Problems of Malaria Control in Tropical Africa," *British Medical Journal*, vol. 1, no. 4855 (23 January 1954), 169–174.

Bruce-Chwatt, L. J. "Chemotherapy in Relation to Possibilities of Malaria Eradication in Tropical Africa," *Bulletin of the World Health Organization*, vol. 15, nos. 3–5 (1956), 852.

Bruce-Chwatt, L. J. "A Longitudinal Study of Natural Malaria Infection in a Group of West African Adults. I," *West African Medical Journal*, vol. 12 (1963), 141–173.

Bruce-Chwatt, L. J. "A Longitudinal Survey of Natural Malaria Infection in a Group of West African Adults. II," *West African Medical Journal*, vol. 12 (1963), 199–217.

Bruce-Chwatt. L. J. "Movements of Populations in Relation to Communicable Disease in Africa," *East African Medical Journal*, vol. 45, no. 5 (1968), 266–275.

Bruce-Chwatt, L. J. "Malaria in Mauritius – As Dead as the Dodo," *Bulletin of the New York Academy of Medicine*, vol. 50, no. 10 (November 1974), 1069–1080.

Bruce-Chwatt, L. J. "Resurgence of Malaria and Its Control," *Journal of Tropical Medicine and Hygiene*, vol. 77, no. 4 (1974), 62–66.

Bruce-Chwatt, L. J. "Lessons Learned from Applied Field Research Activities in Africa during the Malaria Eradication Era," *Bulletin of the World Health Organization*, vol. 62, supplement (1984), 19–29.

Bruce-Chwatt, L. J., H. Archibald, R. Elliott, R. A. Fitz-John, and I. A. Balogus. "Ilaro Experimental Malaria Control Scheme: Report on Four Years' Results," *Fifth International Congress on Tropical Medicine and Malaria*, vol. 2 *Communications* (Istanbul, 1953), 54–66.

Bryce, J., J. B. Roungou, P. Nguyen-Dinh, J. F. Naimoli, and J. G. Breman. "Evaluation of National Malaria Control Programmes in Africa," *Bulletin of the World Health Organization*, vol. 72, no. 3 (1994), 371–381.

Buck, A. A. (ed.). *Proceedings of the Conference on Malaria in Africa. Practical Considerations on Malaria Vaccines and Clinical Trials. Washington, DC, USA, December 1–4, 1986* (Washington, DC: American Institute of Biological Sciences, 1987).

Calonne, R. "La malaria dans le Haut-Ituri," *Annales de la Société belge de médecine tropicale*, vol. 15 (1935), 501–520.

Cambournac, F. J. C., A. F. Gándara, A. J. Pena, and W. L. G. Teixeira. "Subsídios Para o Inquérito Malariológico em Angola," *Anais do Instituto de Medicina Tropical*, vol. 12, nos. 1–2 (1955), 121–153.

Campbell, C. C. "Challenges Facing Antimalarial Therapy in Africa," *Journal of Infectious Diseases*, vol. 163, no. 6 (1991), 1207–1211.

Campbell, J. McP. "Malaria in the Uasin Gishu and Trans-Nzoia," *Kenya and East African Medical Journal*, vol. 6, no. 2 (May 1929), 32–43.

Carlson, D. G. *African Fever: A Study of British Science, Technology, and Politics in West Africa, 1787–1864* (Canton, MA: Science History Publications, 1984).

Carlton, J. M., A. Das, and A. A. Escalante. "Genomics, Population Genetics and Evolutionary History of *Plasmodium vivax*," *Advances in Parasitology*, vol. 81 (2013), 203–222.

Carmouze (Dr.). "La fièvre bilieuse hématurique au Soudan (hivernage 1896)," *Archives de médecine navale*, vol. 67 (1897), 337–356.

Carnevale, P., and J. Mouchet. "Le paludisme en zone de transmission continue en region afrotropicale," *Cahiers ORSTOM*, série Entomologie médicale et Parasitologie, vol. 18, no. 2 (1980), 149–186.

Carnevale, P., and J. Mouchet. "La lutte antivectorielle au Cameroun. Passé-présent-avenir. Réflexions," *Bullétin de la Société de pathologie exotique*, vol. 94, no. 2 (2001), 202–209.

Carnevale, P., V. Robert, C. Boudin, J.-M. Halna, L. Pazart, P. Gazin, A. Richard, and J. Mouchet. "La lutte contre le paludisme par des moustiquaires imprégnées de pyréthrinoides au Burkina Faso," *Bullétin de la Société de pathologie exotique*, vol. 81, no. 5 (1988), 832–846.

Casagrande, R. A. "Colorado Potato Beetle: 125 Years of Mismanagement," *Bulletin of the Entomological Society of America*, vol. 33, no. 3 (1987), 142–150.

Cavalli-Sforza, L. L., P. Menozzi, and A. Piazza. *The History and Geography of Human Genes* (Princeton, NJ: Princeton University Press, 1994).

Chanda, E., J. Hemingway, I. Kleinschmidt, A. M. Rehman, V. Ramdeen, F. N. Phiri, S. Coetzer, D. Mthembu, C. J. Shinondo, E. Chizema-Kawesha, M. Kamuliwo, V. Mukonka, K. S. Baboo, and M. Coleman. "Insecticide Resistance and the Future of Malaria Control in Zambia," *PLOS ONE*, vol. 6, no. 9 (2011), 1–9.

Chanda, E., F. Masaninga, M. Coleman, C. Sikaala, C. Katebe, M. MacDonald, K. S. Baboo, J. Govere, and L. Manga. "Integrated Vector Management: The Zambian Experience," *Malaria Journal*, vol. 7 (2008), no. 194. Available online: http://www.malariajournal.com/content/Pdf/1475-2875-7-164.Pdf

Chandre, F., F. Darier, L. Manga, M. Akogbeto, O. Faye, J. Mouchet, and P. Guillet. "Status of Pyrethroid Resistance in *Anopheles gambiae sensu lato*," *Bulletin of the World Health Organization*, vol. 77, no. 3 (1999), 230–234.

Chataway, J. H. H. "Report on the Malaria Epidemic in the Lumbwa Reserve (August, 1928)," *Kenya and East African Medical Journal*, vol. 5 (1928–1929), 303–309.

Checchi, F., J. Cox, S. Balkan, A. Tamrat, G. Priotto, K. P. Alberti, D. Zurovac, and J.-P. Guthmann. "Malaria Epidemics and Interventions, Kenya, Burundi, Southern Sudan, and Ethiopia, 1999–2004," *Emerging Infectious Diseases*, vol. 12, no. 10 (2006), 1473–1485.

Chima, R. I., C. A. Goodman, and A. Mills. "The Economic Impact of Malaria in Africa: A Critical Review of the Evidence," *Health Policy*, vol. 63, no. 1 (2003), 17–36.

Ch'ng, J. H., L. Renia, F. Nosten, and K. S. W. Tan. "Can We Teach an Old Drug New Tricks?," *Trends in Parasitology*, vol. 28, no. 6 (2012), 220–224.

Christophers, S. R. "The Mechanism of Immunity against Malaria in Communities Living under Hyper-endemic Conditions," *Indian Journal of Medical Research*, vol. 12, no. 2 (1924), 273–294.

Christophers, S. R., and J. W. W. Stephens. "The Segregation of Europeans," in *Reports to the Malarial Committee of the Royal Society*, third series (London: Harrison and Sons, 1900), 21–24.

Christophers, S. R., and J. W. W. Stephens. "The Native as the Prime Agent in the Malarial Infection of the Europeans," in *Further Reports to the Malaria Committee of the Royal Society* (London: Harrison and Sons, 1900), 3–19.

Cleaver, H. "Malaria and the Political Economy of Public Health," *International Journal of Health Services*, vol. 7, no. 4 (1977), 557–579.

Clyde, D. F. "Suppression of Malaria in Tanzania with the Use of Medicated Salt," *Bulletin of the World Health Organization*, vol. 35, no. 6 (1966), 962–968.

Clyde, D. F. *Malaria in Tanzania* (London: Oxford University Press, 1967).

Clyde, D. F. "Recent Trends in the Epidemiology and Control of Malaria," *Epidemiologic Reviews*, vol. 9 (1987), 219–243.

Cockburn, R., P. N. Newton, E. K. Agyarko, D. Akunyili, and N. J. White. "The Global Threat of Counterfeit Drugs: Why Industry and Governments Must Communicate the Dangers," *PLOS Medicine*, vol. 2, no. 4 (2005), 302–308.

Cohen, J. M., D. L. Smith, C. Cotter, A. Ward, G. Yamey, O. J. Sabot, and B. Moonen. "Malaria Resurgence: A Systematic Review and Assessment of Its Causes," *Malaria Journal*, vol. 11 (2012), no. 122. Available online: http://www.malariajournal.com/content/11/1/122

Colbourne, M. *Malaria in Africa* (London: Oxford University Press, 1966).

Colbourne, M. J. "Malaria in Gold Coast Students on Their Return from the United Kingdom," *Transactions of the Royal Society for Tropical Medicine and Hygiene*, vol. 49, no. 5 (1955), 483–487.

Colbourne, M. J. "The Effect of Malaria Suppression in a Group of Accra School Children," *Transactions of the Royal Society for Tropical Medicine and Hygiene*, vol. 49, no. 4 (1955), 356–369.

Colbourne, M. J., and G. M. Edington. "Mortality from Malaria in Accra," *Journal of Tropical Medicine and Hygiene*, vol. 57, no. 9 (1954), 203–210.

Colbourne, M. J., and F. N. Wright. "Malaria in the Gold Coast," *West African Medical Journal*, vol. 4, no. 1 (1955), 3–17 and vol. 4, no. 4 (1955), 161–174.

Collins, W. E., and G. M. Jeffery. "*Plasmodium ovale*: Parasite and Disease," *Clinical Microbiology Reviews*, vol. 18, no. 3 (2005), 570–581.

Collins, W. E., and G. M. Jeffery. "*Plasmodium malariae*: Parasite and Disease," *Clinical Microbiology Reviews*, vol. 20, no. 4 (2005), 579–592.

Colombo, U. "Prophylaxie individuelle antimalarienne chez Européens d'Élisabethville," *Annales de la Société belge de médecine tropicale*, vol. 11, no. 4 (1931), 373–385.

Cook, G. C. "Charles Wilberforce Daniels, FRCP (1862–1927): Underrated Pioneer of Tropical Medicine," *Acta Tropica*, vol. 81, no. 3 (2002), 237–250.

Corre, A. "Compte-rendu d'ouvrages: Traité des fièvres palustres," *Archives de médecine navale*, vol. 41 (1884), 417–419.

Cowan, J. M. "Cinchona in the Empire," *Empire Forestry Journal*, vol. 8, no. 1 (1929), 45–53.

Coz, J., and J. Hamon. "Importance pratique de la résistance aux insecticides en Afrique au sud du Sahara pour L'éradication du paludisme dans ce continent," *Cahiers O. R. S. T. O. M.*, *Série Entomologie Médicale*, no. 1 (1963), 27–37.

Cross, D. K. *Health in Africa: A Medical Handbook for European Travellers and Residents, Embracing a Study of Malarial Fever as It Is Found in British Central Africa* (London: James Nisbet & Co., Ltd., 1897).

Crosse, W. H. *Notes on the Malarial Fevers Met with on the River Niger (West Africa)* (London: Simpkin, Marshall, Hamilton, Kent and H. H. G. Gratton, 1892).

Crosse, W. H. *Hints, Suggestions and Medical Notes for Those Traveling in West Africa* (London: F. R. B. Parmeter, 1903).

Cowan, J. M. "Cinchona in the Empire," *Empire Forestry Journal*, vol. 8, no. 1 (1929), 45–53.

Cox-Singh, J., and B. Singh. "Knowlesi Malaria: Newly Emergent and of Public Health Importance?," *Trends in Parasitology*, vol. 24, no. 9 (2008), 406–410.

Culleton, R., and R. Carter. "African *Plasmodium vivax*: Distribution and Origins," *International Journal for Parasitology*, vol. 42 (2012), 1091–1097.

Curtin, P. D. *The Image of Africa: British Ideas and Action, 1780–1850* (Madison: University of Wisconsin Press, 1964).

Curtin, P. D. "Epidemiology and the Slave Trade," *Political Science Quarterly*, vol. 83, no. 2 (1968), 190–216.

Curtin, P. D. *The Atlantic Slave Trade: A Census* (Madison: University of Wisconsin Press, 1969).

Curtin, P. D. "Medical Knowledge and Urban Planning in Colonial Tropical Africa," *American Historical Review*, vol. 90, no. 3 (1985), 594–613.

Curtin, P. D. *Death by Migration: Europe's Encounter with the Tropical World in the Nineteenth Century* (New York: Cambridge University Press, 1989).

Curtin, P. D. *Disease and Empire: The Health of European Troops in the Conquest of Africa* (New York: Cambridge University Press, 1998).

Curtin, P. D., S. Feierman, L. Thompson, and J. Vansina. *African History: From Earliest Times to Independence* (New York: Longman, 1995).

Curtis, C., C. Maxwell, M. Lemnge, W. L. Kilama, R. W. Steketee, W. A. Hawley, Y. Bergevin, C. C. Campbell, J. Sachs, A. Teklehaimanot, S. Ochola, H. Guyatt, and R. W. Snow. "Scaling-up Coverage with Insecticide-Treated Nets against Malaria in Africa: Who Should Pay?," *The Lancet Infectious Diseases*, vol. 3, no. 5 (2002), 304–307.

Curtis, C. F. "Restoration of Malaria Control in the Madagascar Highlands by DDT Spraying," *American Journal of Tropical Medicine and Hygiene*, vol. 66, no. 1 (2002), 1.

Curtis, C. F., and A. E. P. Mnzava. "Comparison of House Spraying and Insecticide-treated Nets for Malaria Control," *Bulletin of the World Health Organization*, vol. 78, no. 12 (2000), 1389–1400.

D'Alessandro, U., B. Olaleye, P. Langerock, M. K. Aikins, M. C. Thomson, M. K. Cham, B. M. Greenwood, W. McGuire, S. Bennett, M. K. Cham, and B. A. Cham. "Mortality and Morbidity from Malaria in Gambian Children after Introduction of an Impregnated Bednet Programme," *The Lancet*, vol. 345, no. 8948 (25 February 1995), 479–483.

Dalrymple, D. G. *Artemisia annua, Artemisinin, ACTs, and Malaria Control in Africa: Tradition, Science, and Public Policy*, 4th edition (Washington, DC: Politics and Prose Bookstore, 2013).

Daniel, H. I., and N. B. Molta. "Efficacy of Chloroquine in the Treatment of Malaria in Children under Five Years in Baissa (Gongola State, Nigeria)," *Annals of Tropical Medicine and Parasitology*, vol. 83, no. 4 (1989), 331–338.

Daniels, C. W. "Prophylaxis," in *Reports to the Malaria Committee of the Royal Society*, third series (London: Harrison and Sons, 1900), 37–44.

Daniels, C. W. "Notes on 'Blackwater Fever' in British Central Africa," in *Reports to the Malaria Committee of the Royal Society*, fifth series (London: Harrison and Sons, 1901), 44–79.

David, P. *Les navétanes: Histoire des migrants saisonniers de l'arachide en Sénégambie des origins à nos jours* (Dakar: Nouvelles Éditions Africaines, 1980).

Davidson, G. "Field Trials with "Gammexane" as a Means of Malaria Control by Adult Mosquito Destruction in Sierra Leone," *Annals of Tropical Medicine*, vol. 41, no. 2 (1947), 178–209.

Davidson, G. "A Field Study on 'Gammexane' and Malaria Control in the Belgian Congo. II. The Effect of the Spraying of Houses with 'Gammexane' on the Mosquito Population and on the Malaria Incidence in Children," *Annals of Tropical Medicine and Parasitology*, vol. 44, no. 1 (1950), 1–26.

Davidson, G. "Results of Recent Experiments on the Use of DDT and BHC against Adult Mosquitos at Taveta, Kenya," *Bulletin of the World Health Organization*, vol. 4, no. 3 (1951), 329–332.

Davidson, G. "Experiments on the Effect of Residual Insecticides in Houses against *Anopheles gambiae* and *A. Funestus*," *Bulletin of Entomological Research*, vol. 44, no. 2 (1953), 231–254.

Davidson, G., and C.C. Draper. "Field Studies of Some of the Basic Factors Concerned in the Transmission of Malaria," *Transactions of the Royal Society of Tropical Medicine and Hygiene*, vol. 46, no. 6 (1953), 522–535.

Davies, K.G. "The Living and the Dead: White Mortality in West Africa, 1684–1732," in Stanley L. Engerman and Eugene D. Genovese (eds.), *Race and Slavery in the Western Hemisphere: Quantitative Studies* (Princeton, NJ: Princeton University Press, 1975), 83–98.

Day, K.P., J.C. Koella, S. Nee, S. Gupta, and A.F. Read. "Population Genetics and Dynamics of *Plasmodium falciparum*: An Ecological View," *Parasitology*, vol. 104, issue S1 (1992), s35–s52.

de Boer, H.S. "Malaria and Its Control on Mombasa Island," *Kenya and East African Medical Journal*, vol. 5, no. 1 (1928), 2–11.

de Boer, H.S. "Anti Malarial Measures in Towns," *Kenya and East African Medical Journal*, vol. 7, no. 9 (1930), 256–270.

Delacollette, C., P. Van der Stuyft, K. Molima, C. Delacollette-Lebrun, and M. Wery. "Etude de la mortalité globale et de la mortalité lieé au paludisme dans le Kivu montagneux, Zaire," *Révue d'epidemiologie et de la santé publique*, vol. 37, no. 2 (1989), 161–166.

De Meillon, B. "The Control of Malaria in South Africa by Measures Directed against the Adult Mosquitoes in Habitations," *Quarterly Bulletin of the Health Organisation of the League of Nations*, vol. 5 (1936), 134–137.

De Meillon, B. "Species and Varieties of Malaria Vectors in Africa and Their Bionomics," *Bulletin of the World Health Organization*, vol. 4, no. 3 (1951), 419–441.

de Mello, J.P. "Some Aspects of Malaria in Kenya," *East African Medical Journal*, vol. 24, no. 3 (March 1947), 112–126.

de Mello, J.P. "Survey of Malaria among the Indigenous Population in the Highlands of Kenya: With Reference to Hyperendemic Areas," *East African Medical Journal*, vol. 28, no. 11 (1951), 465–472.

De Smet, M.P. "Traitement d'attaque des anémies-oedèmes graves par transfusions fractionnées chez les enfants sevrés," *Annales de la Société belge de médecine tropicale*, vol. 34 (1954), 155–169.

Desowitz, R.S. *New Guinea Tapeworms and Jewish Grandmothers: Tales of Parasites and People* (New York: W.W. Norton, 1981).

Dixon, D.S. "Paludrine (Proguanil) as a Malarial Prophylactic Amongst African Labour in Kenya," *East African Medical Journal*, vol. 27, no. 3 (1950), 127–130.

Dodge, C.P., and P.D. Wiebe. *Crisis in Uganda: The Breakdown of Health Services* (Oxford: Pergamon Press, 1985).

Dolo, G., O.J.T. Briët, A. Dao, S.F. Traoré, M. Bouaré, N. Sogoba, O. Niaré, M. Bagayogo, D. Sangaré, T. Teuscher, and Y.T. Touré. "Malaria Transmission in Relation to Rice Cultivation in the Irrigated Sahel of Mali," *Acta Tropica*, vol. 89, no. 2 (2004), 147–159.

Dondorp, A. M., S. Yeung, L. White, C. Nguon, N. P. J. Day, D. Socheat, and
L. von Seidlein. "Artemisinin Resistance: Current Status and Scenarios for
Containment," *Nature Reviews Microbiology*, vol. 8, no. 4 (2010), 272–280.

Doolan, D. L., C. Dobaño, and J. K. Baird. "Acquired Immunity to Malaria,"
Clinical Microbiology Reviews, vol. 22, no. 1 (2009), 13–36.

Dowling, M. A. C. "An Experiment in the Eradication of Malaria in Mauritius,"
Bulletin of the World Health Organization, vol. 4 (1951), 443–461.

Dowling, M. A. C. "The Malaria Eradication Scheme in Mauritius," *British
Medical Bulletin*, vol. 8, no. 1 (1951), 72–75.

Dowling, M. A. C. "Malaria Control in Mauritius," *British Medical Bulletin*, vol. 9
(9 August 1952), 309–312.

Dowling, M. A. C. "Control of Malaria in Mauritius: Eradication of *Anopheles
funestus* and *Aedes aegypti*," *Transactions of the Royal Society of Tropical
Medicine and Hygiene*, vol. 47, no. 3 (1953), 177–198.

Draper, C. C., G. Brubaker, A. Geser, V. A. E. B. Kilimali, and W. H. Wernsdorfer.
"Serial Studies on the Evolution of Chloroquine Resistance in an Area of East
Africa Receiving Intermittent Malaria Chemosuppression," *Bulletin of the
World Health Organization*, vol. 63, no. 1 (1985), 109–118.

Draper, C. C., J. L. M. Lelijveld, Y. G. Matola, and G. B. White. "Malaria in the
Pare Area of Tanzania. IV. Malaria in the Human Population 11 Years after
the Suspension of Residual Insecticide Spraying, with Special Reference to the
Serological Findings," *Transactions of the Royal Society of Tropical Medicine
and Hygiene*, vol. 66, no. 6 (1972), 905–912.

Draper, C. C., and A. Smith. "Malaria in the Pare Area of Tanzania. Part 2. Effects
of Three Years' Spraying of Parts with Dieldrin," *Transactions of the Royal
Society of Tropical Medicine and Hygiene*, vol. 54, no. 4 (1960), 342–357.

Dua, V. K. A. C. Pandey, K. Raghavendra, A. Gupta, T. Sharma, and A. P. Dash.
"Larvicidal Activity of Neem Oil (*Azadirachta indica*) Formulation against
Mosquitoes," *Malaria Journal*, vol. 8 (2009). Available online: http://www.
malariajournal.com/content/8/1/124

Dugbatey, K. "National Health Policies: Sub-Saharan African Case Studies (1980–
1990)," *Social Science and Medicine*, vol. 49, no. 2 (1999), 223–239.

Dumett, R. E. "The Campaign against Malaria and the Expansion of Scientific
Medical and Sanitary Services in British West Africa, 1898–1910," *African
Historical Studies*, vol. 1, no. 2 (1968), 153–197.

Duren, A. "Contribution à l'étude du paludisme endémique au Congo Belge,
district du Kwango," *Annales de la Société belge de médecine tropicale*,
vol. 20, no. 3 (1930), 265–277.

Duren, A. "Un essai d'étude d'ensemble du paludisme au Congo Belge," *Institut
Royal Colonial Belge, Section des sciences naturelles et médicales. Mémoires*,
vol. 5, no. 5 (1937), 1–87.

Dutton, J. E. *Report of the Malaria Expedition to the Gambia (1902)*. Memoir X
(London: Longmans, Green, & Co. for the University Press of Liverpool, 1903).

East African Institute of Malaria and Vector-Borne Diseases in Collaboration with
Colonial Pesticides Research Unit. *Report on the Pare-Taveta Scheme 1954–
1959* (Dar es Salaam: Government Printer, 1960).

Echenberg, M. *Africa in the Time of Cholera: A History of Pandemics from 1817 to the Present* (New York: Cambridge University Press, 2011).

Eckart, W. U. "Malaria and Colonialism in the German Colonies New Guinea and the Cameroons. Research, Control, Thoughts of Eradication," *Parassitologia*, vol. 40 (1998), 83–90.

Ecker, A., A. M. Lehane, J. Clain, and D. A. Fidock. "PfCRT and Its Role in Antimalarial Drug Resistance," *Trends in Parasitology*, vol. 28, no. 11 (2012), 504–514.

Eddey, L. G. "Spray Killing of Mosquitoes in Houses, A Contribution to Malaria Control on the Gold Coast," *Transactions of the Royal Society of Tropical Medicine and Hygiene*, vol. 38, no. 3 (1944), 167–197.

Edington, G. M. "Pathology of Malaria in West Africa," *British Medical Journal*, vol. 1, no. 5542 (25 March 1967), 715–718.

Ehret, C. *The Civilizations of Africa: A History to 1800* (Charlottesville: University of Virginia Press, 2002).

Eisele, T. P., D. A. Larsen, N. Walker, R. E. Cibulskis, J. O. Yukich, C. M. Zikusooka, and R. W. Steketee. "Estimates of Child Deaths Prevented from Malaria Prevention Scale-up in Africa 2001–2010," *Malaria Journal*, vol. 11 (2012), no. 93. Available online: http://www.malariajournal.com/content/11/1/93/

Elliott, R. "The Influence of Vector Behavior on Malaria Transmission," *American Journal of Tropical Medicine and Hygiene*, vol. 21, no. 5 (1972), 755–763.

Escudie, A., J. Hamon, J.-H. Ricosse, and A. Chartol. "Résultats de deux années de chimioprophylaxie antipaludique en milieu rural africain dans la zone pilote de Bobo Dioulasso (Haute Volta)," *Médecine tropicale*, vol. 21 (1961), 689–728.

Ewers, W. "Robert Koch, His Work in New Guinea, and His Contribution to Malariology," *Papua New Guinea Medical Journal*, vol. 15, no. 2 (1972), 117–124.

Falcot, J., F. Meignan, J. Thierry, and J. L. Perret. "Chimioresistance du *Plasmodium falciparum* en Afrique Centrale," *Médecine et maladies infectieuses*, vol. 17, no. 3 (1987), 133.

Feacham, R., and O. Sabot. "A New Global Malaria Eradication Strategy," *The Lancet*, vol. 371 (2008) 1633–1635.

Feacham, R. G. A., A. A. Phillips, and G. A. Targett (eds.). *Shrinking the Malaria Map: A Prospectus for Malaria Elimination* (San Francisco: The Global Health Group, 2009).

Fendall, N. R. E., and J. G. Grounds. "The Incidence and Epidemiology of Disease in Kenya. Part II. Some Important Communicable Diseases," *Journal of Tropical Medicine and Hygiene*, vol. 68 (1965), 113–120.

Feuillat, F., M. Parent, E. M. E. Peeters, and I. H. Vincke. "Progrès récents dans la lutte anti-malarienne au Katanga," *Annales de la Société belge de médecine tropicale*, vol. 33 (1953), 621–674.

Fieldhouse, D. K. *Black Africa, 1945–1980: Economic Decolonization and Arrested Development* (London: Unwin Hyman, 1986).

Fleischer, B. "Editorial: 100 Years Ago: Giemsa's Solution for Staining of Plasmodia," *Tropical Medicine and International Health*, vol. 9, no. 7 (2004), 755–756.

Fletcher, T. E., J. M. Press, and D. Bagster Wilson. "Exposure of Spray-men to Dieldrin in Residual Spraying," *Bulletin of the World Health Organization*, vol. 20, no. 1 (1959), 15–25.

Foley, E. E. *Your Pocket Is What Cures You: The Politics of Health in Senegal* (New Brunswick, NJ: Rutgers University Press, 2010).

Foll, C. V., C. P. Pant, and P. E. Lietaert. "A Large-Scale Field Trial with Dichlorvos as a Residual Fumigant Insecticide in Northern Nigeria," *Bulletin of the World Health Organization*, vol. 32, no. 4 (1965), 531–550.

Fontaine, R. E., J. H. Pull, D. Payne, G. D. Pradhan, G. P, Goshi, J. A. Pearson, M. K. Thymakis, and M. W. R. Camacho. "Evaluation of Fenitrothion for the Control of Malaria," *Bulletin of the World Health Organization*, vol. 56, no. 3 (1978), 445–452.

Foster, S. D. "Pricing, Distribution, and Use of Antimalarial Drugs," *Bulletin of the World Health Organization*, vol. 69, no. 3 (1991), 349–363.

Frenkel, S., and J. Western. "Pretext or Prophylaxis? Racial Segregation and Malarial Mosquitos in a British Tropical Colony: Sierra Leone," *Annals of the Association of American Geographers*, vol. 78, no. 2 (1988), 211–228.

Gabaldón, A. "Global Eradication of Malaria: Changes of Strategy and Future Outlook," *American Journal of Tropical Medicine and Hygiene*, vol. 18. no. 5 (1969), 641–656.

Garenne, M., and E. Gakusi. "Health Transitions in Sub-Saharan Africa: Overview of Mortality Trends in Children under 5 Years Old (1950–2000)," *Bulletin of the World Health Organization*, vol. 84, no. 6 (2006), 470–478.

Garnham, P. C. C. "Malaria in Kisumu, Kenya Colony," *Journal of Tropical Medicine and Hygiene*, vol. 32 (1929), 207–231.

Garnham, P. C. C. "Hyperendemic Malaria in a Native Reserve of Kenya and the Influence upon Its Course of Atebrin and Plasmoquine," *Transactions of the Royal Society of Tropical Medicine and Hygiene*, vol. 29, no. 2 (1935), 167–186.

Garnham, P. C. C. "Malaria in East Africa," a letter to the editor, *Transactions of the Royal Society of Tropical Medicine and Hygiene*, vol. 33, no. 1 (1939), 132–133.

Garnham, P. C. C. "Malaria Epidemics at Exceptionally High Altitudes in Kenya," *British Medical Journal*, vol. 2, no. 4410 (14 July 1945), 45–47.

Garnham, P. C. C. "Malarial Immunity in Africans: Effects in Infancy and Early Childhood," *Annals of Tropical Medicine and Parasitology*, vol. 43, no. 1 (1947), 47–61.

Garnham, P. C. C. "The Incidence of Malaria at High Altitudes," *Journal of the National Malaria Society*, vol. 7, no. 4 (1948), 275–284.

Garnham, P. C. C. "Modern Concepts in Malaria Control," *Journal of the Royal Sanitary Institute*, vol. 69, no. 5 (1949), 617–625.

Garnham, P. C. C. "Malaria in the African Child," *East African Medical Journal*, vol. 31, no. 4 (1954), 155–159.

Garnham, P. C. C. "The Changing Pattern of Disease in East Africa," *East African Medical Journal*, vol. 45, no. 10 (1968), 641–650.

Garnham, P. C. C. "DDT versus Malaria, Kenya 1946 – Commentary on a Film," in E. E. Sabben-Clare, D. J. Bradley, and K. Kirkwood (eds.), *Health in Tropical Africa during the Colonial Period* (Oxford: Clarendon Press, 1980), 63–66.

Garnham, P. C. C., and J. O. Harper, "The Control of Rural Malaria by Pyrethrum Dusting," *East African Medical Journal*, vol. 21 (1944), 310–319.

Garnham, P. C. C., D. B. Wilson, and M. E. Wilson. "Malaria in Kigezi, Uganda," *Journal of Tropical Medicine and Hygiene*, vol. 51, no. 8 (1948), 156–159.

Gazin, P., M. Cot, V. Robert, and D. Bonnet. "La perception du paludisme en Afrique au sud du Sahara," *Annales de la Société belge de la médecine tropicale*, vol. 68 (1988), 1–3.

Gazin, P., C. Freier, P. Turk, B. Gineste, and P. Carnevale. "Le paludisme chez les employés d'une enterprise industrielle africaine (Bobo Dioulasso, Burkina Faso)," *Annales de la Societé belge de médecine tropicale*, vol. 68, no. 4 (1988), 285–292.

Gelfand, M. *Tropical Victory: An Account of the Influence of Medicine on the History of Southern Rhodesia* (Cape Town: Juta & Co., Ltd, 1953).

Gelfand, M. *Lakeside Pioneers: Socio-Medical Study of Nyasaland (1875–1920)* (Oxford: Basil Blackwell, 1964).

Gelfand, M. *Rivers of Death in Africa* (London: Oxford University Press, 1964).

Gianotti, R. L., A. Bomblies, M. Dafalla, I. Issa-Arzika, J. -B. Duchemin, and E. A. B. Eltahir. "Efficacy of Local Neem Extracts for Sustainable Malaria Vector Control in an African Village," *Malaria Journal*, vol. 7 (2008). Available online: http://www.malariajournal/content/7/1/138

Gibson, F. D. "Malaria Parasite Survey of Some Areas in the Southern Cameroons under United Kingdom Administration," *West African Medical Journal*, vol. 7 (1958), 170–178.

Giglioli, G. "Malaria Control in British Guiana," *Bulletin of the World Health Organization*, vol. 11 (1954), 849–853.

Giglioli, G. *Demerara Doctor: An Early Success against Malaria. The Autobiography of a Self-Taught Physician, George Giglioli (1897–1975)* (London: Smith-Gordon, 2006).

Giles, Lieut.-Colonel. *General Sanitation and Anti-Malarial Measures in Sekondi, the Goldfields and Kumassi* (London: Williams & Norgate for the University of Liverpool Press, 1905).

Giles-Vernick, T., A. Traoré, and S. B. Sirima. "Malaria, Environmental Change, and an Historical Epidemiology of Childhood 'Cold Fevers': Popular Interpretations from Southwestern Burkina Faso," *Health and Place*, vol. 17, no. 6 (2011), 836–842.

Gilles, H. M., and R. G. Hendrickse. "Nephrosis in Nigerian Children. Role of *Plasmodium malariae*, and Effect of Antimalarial Treatment," *British Medical Journal*, vol. 2 (6 July 1963), 27–31.

Gilly, C. "Activité du service d'hygiène de la circonscription de Dakar pendant l'hivernage 1933 (1er juin au 1er décembre)," *Bullétin de la Société de pathologie exotique*, vol. 27, no. 1 (1934), 87–93.

Gilroy, A. B. *Malaria Control by Coastal Swamp Drainage in West Africa* (Calcutta: Ross Institute, LSHTM, 1948).

Gilson, L., and A. Mills. "Health Sector Reforms in Sub-Saharan Africa: Lessons of the Last 10 Years," *Health Policy*, vol. 32, nos. 1–3 (1995), 215–243.

Gordon, R. M., and T. H. Davey. "*P. malariae* in Freetown, Sierra Leone," *Annals of Tropical Medicine and Parasitology*, vol. 26 (1932), 65–84.

Gordon, R. M., and T. H. Davey. "A Further Note on the Increase of *P. malariae* in Freetown, Sierra Leone," *Annals of Tropical Medicine and Parasitology*, vol. 27 (1933), 53–55.

Gordon, R. M., and G. Macdonald. "The Transmission of Malaria in Sierra Leone," *Annals of Tropical Medicine and Parasitology*, vol. 24, no. 1 (1930), 69–80.

Gosling, R. D., I. Carniero, and D. Chandromohan. "Intermittent Preventive Treatment of Malaria in Infants: How Does It Work, and Where Will It Work?," *Tropical Medicine and International Health*, vol. 14, no. 9 (2009), 1003–1010.

Gottlieb, A. *The Afterlife Is Where We Come from: The Culture of Infancy in West Africa* (Chicago: University of Chicago Press, 2004).

Gramont, J. -L. "Le paludisme," *Marchés tropicaux* (novembre 1947), 1679–1683.

Greenwood, B. M. "The Impact of Malaria Chemoprophylaxis on the Immune Status of Africans," *Bulletin of the World Health Organization*, vol. 62, supplement (1984), 69–75.

Greenwood, B. M. "Summary and Conclusions," *Transactions of the Royal Society of Tropical Medicine and Hygiene*, vol. 87, supplement 2 (1993), 59–60.

Greenwood, B. M. "The Epidemiology of Malaria," *Annals of Tropical Medicine and Parasitology*, vol. 91, no. 7 (1997), 763–769.

Greenwood, B. M., and H. Pickering. "A Malaria Control Trial Using Insecticide-Treated Bed Nets and Targeted Chemoprophylaxis in a Rural Area of The Gambia, West Africa. 1. A Review of the Epidemiology and Control of Malaria in The Gambia, West Africa," *Transactions of the Royal Society of Tropical Medicine and Hygiene*, vol. 87, supplement 2 (1993), 3–11.

Griffin, J. T., T. D. Hollingsworth, L. C. Okell, T. S. Churcher, M. White, W. Hinsley, T. Bousema, C. J. Drakeley, N. M. Ferguson, M. -G. Basáñez, and A. C. Ghani. "Reducing *Plasmodium falciparum* Malaria Transmission in Africa: A Model-Based Evaluation of Intervention Strategies," *PLOS Medicine*, vol. 7, no. 8 (2010), 1–17, e1000324.

Guèye, I. "Lutte antipaludique et politique de prééradication au Sénégal," *Bullétin de la Société médicale d'Afrique Noire*, vol. 12 no. 2 (1965), 47–49.

Gupta, S., R. W. Snow, C. A. Donnelly, K. Marsh, and C. Newbold. "Immunity to Non-Cerebral Severe Malaria Is Acquired after One or Two Infections," *Nature Medicine*, vol. 5, no. 3 (1999), 340–343.

Guyatt, H. L., S. A. Ocholo, and R. W. Snow. "Too Poor to Pay: Charging for Insecticide Treated Bed Nets in Highland Kenya," *Tropical Medicine and International Health*, vol. 7, no. 10 (2002), 846–850.

Guyatt, H. L., and R. W. Snow. "Malaria in Pregnancy as an Indirect Cause of Infant Mortality in Sub-Saharan Africa," *Transactions of the Royal Society of Tropical Medicine and Hygiene*, vol. 95 (2001), 569–576.

Hall, S. A., and N. E. Wilks. "A Trial of Chloroquine-Medicated Salt for Malaria Suppression in Uganda," *American Journal of Tropical Medicine and Hygiene*, vol. 16, no. 4 (1967), 429–442.

Hamon, J., B. Dedewanou, and M. Eyraud. "Etudes entomologiques sur la transmission du paludisme humain dans une zone forestière africaine, la région de Man, République de Côte d'Ivoire," *Bullétin de l'Institut Fondamental d'Afrique Noire*, vol. 24, no. 3, series A (1962), 854–879.

Hamon, J., and J. Mouchet. "La résistance aux insecticides chez les insects d'importance médicale. Méthodes d'étude et situation en Afrique au sud du Sahara," *Médecine tropicale*, vol. 21, no. 5 (1961), 565–596.

Hamon, J., J. Mouchet, and G. Chauvet. "Bilan de quatorze années de lutte contre le paludisme dans les pays francophones d'Afrique tropicale et à Madagascar. Considérations sur la persistence de la transmission et perspectives d'avenir," *Bullétin de la Société de pathologie exotique*, vol. 56, no. 5 (sept-oct 1963), 933–971.

Harrison, G. *Mosquitoes, Malaria & Man: A History of the Hostilities Since 1880* (New York: E. P. Dutton, 1978).

Harverson, G., and M. E. Wilson. "Assessment of Current Malarial Endemicity in Bathurst, Gambia," *West African Medical Journal*, vol. 17, no. 3 (1968), 63–67.

Harwin, R. M. "Increase of Malaria in Zimbabwe Rhodesia: Fact or Fiction?," *The Zimbabwe Rhodesia Science News*, vol. 13, no. 8 (August 1979), 177–178 and 189.

Hay, S. I., C. A. Guerra, A. J. Tatem, P. M. Atkinson, and R. W. Snow. "Tropical Infectious Diseases: Urbanization, Malaria Transmission, and the Disease Burden in Africa," *Nature Reviews Microbiology*, vol. 3 (January 2005), 81–90.

Hayes, Jr., W. J. "Dieldrin Poisoning in Man," *Public Health Reports*, vol. 72, no. 12 (1957), 1087–1091.

Hayes, W. S. "The Malaria Epidemic," *East African Medical Journal*, vol. 7 (1940), 216–220.

Hedman, P., J. Brohult, J. Forslund, V. Sirleaf, and E. Bengtsson. "A Pocket of Controlled Malaria in a Holoendemic Region of West Africa," *Annals of Tropical Medicine and Parasitology*, vol. 73, no. 4 (1979), 317–325.

Henderson, D. A. *Smallpox: The Death of a Disease* (Amherst, NY: Prometheus Books, 2009).

Henderson, L. H. "Prophylaxis of Malaria in the Sudan," *Transactions of the Royal Society of Tropical Medicine and Hygiene*, vol. 38 (1934), 157.

Hendrickse, R. G. et al. "Malaria in Early Childhood," *Annals of Tropical Medicine and Parasitology*, vol. 65 (1971), 1–20.

Hill, P. *Development Economics on Trial: The Anthropological Case for a Prosecution* (Cambridge, 1986).

Hocking, K. S. "Residual Action of DDT against A. gambiae and A. funestus," *Transactions of the Royal Society for Tropical Medicine and Hygiene*, vol. 40, no. 5 (1947), 589–601.

Holstein, M. H. "Note sur l'épidémiologie du paludisme en Afrique-Occidentale Française," *Bulletin of the World Health Organization*," vol. 4, no. 3 (1951), 463–473.

Holstein, M. H. *Biology of Anopheles gambiae. Research in French West Africa.* World Health Organization monograph no. 9 (Geneva, WHO, 1954).

Hongoro, C., and B. McPake. "How to Bridge the Gap in Human Resources for Health," *The Lancet*, vol. 364 (16 October 2004), 1451–1456.

Hotez, P. J., and D. H. Molyneux. "Tropical Anemia: One of Africa's Great Killers and a Rationale for Linking Malaria and Neglected Tropical Disease Control to Achieve a Common Goal," *PLOS Neglected Tropical Diseases*, vol. 2, no. 7 (2008), e270.

Howard, L. O. *Mosquitoes* (New York: McClure, Phillips & Co., 1901).

Humphreys, M. "Kicking a Dying Dog: DDT and the Demise of Malaria in the American South," *Isis*, vol. 87, no. 1 (1996), 1–17.

Hsu, E. "The History of Qing Hao in the Chinese Materia Medica," *Transactions of the Royal Society of Tropical Medicine and Hygiene*, vol. 100 (2006), 505–508.

Hsu, E. "Reflections on the 'Discovery' of the Antimalarial Qinghao," *British Journal of Clinical Pharmacology*, vol. 61, no. 6 (2006), 666–670.

Hughes, C. C., and J. M. Hunter. "Disease and 'Development' in Africa," *Social Science and Medicine*, vol. 3 (1970), 443–493.

Ijumba, J. N., and S. W. Lindsay. "Impact of Irrigation on Malaria in Africa: Paddies Paradox," *Medical and Veterinary Entomology*, vol. 15, no. 1 (2001), 1–11.

Iliffe, J. *The African AIDS Epidemic: A History* (Athens: Ohio University Press, 2006).

International Cooperation Administration Expert Committee on Malaria. "Report and Recommendations on Malaria: A Summary," *American Journal of Tropical Medicine and Hygiene*, vol. 10, no. 4 (1961), 451–502.

Iroko, A. F. *Une histoire des hommes et des moustiques en Afrique. Côte des Esclaves (XVIème-XIXème siècles)* (Paris: Éditions L'Harmattan, 1994).

Jackson, L. C. "Malaria in Liberian Children and Mothers: Biocultural Perceptions of Illness vs Clinical Evidence of Disease," *Social Science and Medicine*, vol., 20, no. 12 (1985), 1281–1287.

Jaden, J. "Rapport sur la campagne de dédétisation dans le territoire d'Astrida," *Annales de la Société belge de médecine tropicale*, vol. 32, no. 5 (1952), 445–464.

Jaden, J., A. Fain, and H. Rupp. "Lutte anti-malarienne étendue en zone rurale au moyen de D. D. T. à Astrida, Ruanda-Urundi," *Institut Royal Colonial Belge, Section des Sciences Naturelles et Médicales, Mémoires*, vol. 21, fasc. 1 (1952), 1–47.

James, S. P. *Report on a Visit to Kenya and Uganda to Advise on Antimalarial Measures* (London: Crown Agents for the Colonies, 1929).

James, S. P., W. D. Nicol, and P. G. Shute. "A Study of Induced Malignant Tertian Malaria," *Proceedings of the Royal Society of Medicine*, vol. 25, no. 7 (1932), 37–70.

Janssens, P. G., N. Verstraete, and J. Sieniawski. "Essais de chimioprophylaxie antipaludique collective chez les enfants des travailleurs des mines de Kilo," *Annales de la Société belge de médecine tropicale*, vol. 30, no. 2 (1950), 257–286.

Janssens, P. G., N. Verstraete, and J. Sieniawski. "Essais de chimioprophylaxie antipaludique collective chez les enfants des travailleurs des mines de Kilo (Suite)," *Annales de la Société belge de médecine tropicale*, vol. 30, no. 3 (1950), 449–478.

Janssens, P. G., I. H. Vincke, and J. Bafort. "Le paludisme d'Afrique Centrale. Son influence sur la morbidité des enfants," *Bullétin de la Société de pathologie exotique*, vol. 59 (1966), 665.

Janssens, P. G., and M. Wery. "Malaria in Africa South of the Sahara," *Annals of Tropical Medicine and Parasitology*, vol. 81, no. 5 (1987), 487–498.

Jeffrey, G. M. "The Role of Chemotherapy in Malaria Control Through Primary Health Care: Constraints and Future Prospects," *Bulletin of the World Health Organization*, vol. 62, supplement (1984), 49–53.

Jobin, W. R. *Dams and Disease: Ecological Design and Health Impacts of Large Dams, Canals, and Irrigation Systems* (London: E & FN Spon Press, 1999).

Jonchère, H., and R. Pfister. "Enquêtes malariologiques en Haute-Volta, Cote d'Ivoire et Guinée (Janvier-Mars 1951)," *Bullétin de la Société de pathologie exotique*, vol. 44, nos. 11–12 (nov-dec. 1951), 774–786.

Joncour, G. "La lutte contre le paludisme à Madagascar," *Bulletin of the World Health Organization*, vol. 15 (1956), 711–723.

Jones, C. M., H. K. Toé, A. Sanou, M. Namountougou, A. Hughes, A. Diabaté, R. Dabiré, F. Simard, and H. Ranson. "Additional Selection for Insecticide Resistance in Urban Malaria Vectors: DDT Resistance in *Anopheles arabiensis* from Bobo-Dioulasso, Burkina Faso," *PLOS ONE*, vol. 9, no. 9 (2012), 1–9.

Kamat, V. R. "Dying under the Bird's Shadow: Narrative Representations of Degedege and Child Survival among the Zaramo of Tanzania," *Medical Anthropology*, vol. 22, no. 1 (2008), 67–93.

Kaseje, D. C. O. et al. "Usage of Community-Based Chloroquine Treatment for Malaria in Saradidi, Kenya," *Annals of Tropical Medicine and Parasitology*, vol. 81, supplement 1 (1987), 111–115.

Kauntze, W. H., and C. B. Symes. "Anophelines and Malaria at Taveta," *Records of the Medical Research Laboratory, Kenya*, no. 5 (1933).

Keiser, J., J. Utzinger, M. Caldas de Castro, T. A. Smith, M. Tanner, and B. H. Singer. "Urbanization in Sub-Saharan Africa and Implication for Malaria Control," *American Journal of Tropical Medicine and Hygiene*, vol. 71, supplement 2 (2004), 118–127.

Kerbosch, M. "Some Notes on Cinchona Culture and the World Consumption of Quinine," *Bulletin of the Colonial Institute of Amsterdam*, vol. 3, no. 1 (1939), 36–51.

Khromov, A. S. "Epidemiology of Malaria: Specific Features and Control in African Countries," *International Scientific Project on Ecologically Safe Methods for Control of Malaria and Its Vectors* (Moscow, 1980), 72–91.

Killeen, G. F., U. Fillinger, I. Kiche, L. C. Gouagna, and B. G. J. Knols. "Eradication of *Anopheles gambiae* from Brazil: Lessons for Malaria Control in Africa?," *The Lancet Infectious Diseases*, 2 (2002), 618–627.

Kinkela, D. *DDT and the American Century* (Chapel Hill: University of North Carolina Press, 2011).

Kiszewski, A., B. Johns, A. Schapira, C. Delacollette, V. Crowell, T. Tan-Torres, B. Ameneshewa, A. Teklehaimonot, and F. Nafo-Traoré. "Estimated Global Resources Needed to Attain International Malaria Controls," *Bulletin of the World Health Organization*, vol. 85, no. 8 (2007), 623–630.

Kitron, U. "Malaria, Agriculture, and Development: Lessons from Past Campaigns," *International Journal of Health Services*, vol. 17, no. 2 (1987), 295–326.

Kjekshus, H. *Ecology Control and Economic Development in East African History* (Athens: Ohio University Press, 1996).

Kolaczinski, K., J. Kolaczinski, A. Kilian, and S. Meek. "Extension of Indoor Residual Spraying for Malaria Control into High Transmission Settings in Africa," *Transactions of the Royal Society of Tropical Medicine and Hygiene*, vol. 101, 852–853.

Korenromp, E. L., B. G. Williams, S. J. de Vlas, E. Gouws, C. F. Gilks, P. D. Ghys, and B. L. Nahlen. "Malaria Attributable to the HIV-1 Epidemic, Sub-Saharan Africa," *Emerging Infectious Diseases*, vol. 11, no. 9 (2005), 1410–1419.

Kouznetsov, R. L. "Malaria Control by Application of Indoor Spraying of Residual Insecticides in Tropical Africa and Its Impact on Community Health," *Tropical Doctor*, vol. 7 (1977), 81–91.

Kouznetsov, R. L. "Malaria Control: Benefits of Past Activities in Tropical Africa," *WHO Chronicle*, vol. 31 (1977), 98–101.

Kwiatkowski, D., and B. M. Greenwood. "Why Is Malaria Fever Periodic? A Hypothesis," *Parasitology Today*, vol. 5, no. 8 (1989), 264–266.

Laing, A. B. G. "The Impact of Malaria Chemoprophylaxis in Africa with Special Reference to Madagascar, Cameroon, and Senegal," *Bulletin of the World Health Organization*, vol. 62, supplement (1984), 41–48.

Laufer, M. K., and C. V. Plowe. "Withdrawing Antimalarial Drugs: Impact on Parasite Resistance and Implications for Malaria Treatment Policies," *Drug Resistance Updates*, vol. 7 (2004), 279–288.

Laufer, M. K., P. C. Theising, N. D. Eddington, R. Masonga, F. K. Dzinjalamala, S. L. Takala, T. E. Taylor, and C. V. Plowe. "Return of Chloroquine Antimalarial Efficacy in Malawi," *New England Journal of Medicine*, vol. 355, no. 19 (2006), 1959–1966.

Launiala, A., and T. Kulmala. "The Importance of Understanding the Local Context: Women's Perceptions and Knowledge Concerning Malaria in Pregnancy in Rural Malawi," *Acta Tropica*, vol. 98 (2006), 111–117.

Leigh Bennett, H. "Anti-Malarial Drainage," *Kenya and East African Medical Journal*, vol. 7, no. 7 (1930), 190–198.

Le Gouas, J. Le Médicin Commandant. "Mise en place d'un dispositif antipaludique dans la presqu'île de Dakar," *Bullétin Médical de l'Afrique Occidentale Française*, vol. 6, no. 1 (1949), 93–97.

Lengeler, C. "Insecticide-Treated Bed Nets and Curtains for Malaria Control," *Cochrane Database of Systematic Reviews*, issue 2 (2004), 1–47.

Lengeler, C., and R. W. Snow. "From Efficacy to Effectiveness: Insecticide-Treated Bednets in Africa," *Bulletin of the World Health Organization*, vol. 74, no. 3 (1996), 325–332.

Lindblade, K. A., E. D. Walker, A. W. Onapa, J. Katungu, and M. L. Wilson. "Highland Malaria in Uganda: Prospective Analysis of an Epidemic Associated with El Niño," *Transactions of the Royal Society of Tropical Medicine and Hygiene*, vol. 93, no. 5 (1999), 480–487.

Lindsay, S. W., P. L. Alonso, J. R. M. Armestrong Schellenberg, J. Hemingway, J. H. Adiamah, F. C. Shenton, M. Jawara, and B. M. Greenwood. "A Malaria Control Trial Using Insecticide-Treated Bed Nets and Targeted Chemoprophylaxis in a Rural Area of The Gambia, West Africa. 7. Impact of Permethrin-Impregnated Bed Nets on Malaria Vectors," *Transactions of the Royal Society of Tropical Medicine and Hygiene*, vol. 87 (1993), supplement 2, 45–51.

Lindsay, S. W., P. L. Alonso, J. R. M. Armestrong Schellenberg, J. Hemingway, P. J. Thomas, F. C. Shenton, and B. M. Greenwood. "A Malaria Control Trial Using Insecticide-Treated Bed Nets and Targeted Chemoprophylaxis in a Rural Area of The Gambia, West Africa. 3. Entomological Characteristics of the Study

Area," *Transactions of the Royal Society of Tropical Medicine and Hygiene*, vol. 87 (1993), supplement 2, 19–23.

Lindsay, S. W., and W. J. M. Martens. "Malaria in the African Highlands: Past, Present and Future," *Bulletin of the World Health Organization*, vol. 76, no. 1 (1998), 33–45.

Litsios, S. *The Tomorrow of Malaria* (Karori, NZ: Pacific Press, 1996).

Litsios, S. "The Long and Difficult Road to Alma-Ata: A Personal Reflection," *International Journal of Health Services*, vol. 32 (2002), 709–732.

Liu, W., Y. Li, G. H. Learn, R. S. Rudicell, J. D. Robertson, B. F. Keele, J.-B. N. Ndjango, C. M. Sanz, D. B. Morgan, S. Locatelli, M. K. Gonder, P. J. Kranzusch, P. D. Walsh, E. Delaporte, E. Mpoudi-Ngole, A. V. Georgiev, M. N. Muller, G. M. Shaw, M. Peeters, P. M. Sharp, J. C. Rayner, and B. H. Hahn, "Origin of the Human Malaria Parasite *Plasmodium falciparum* in Gorillas," *Nature*, vol. 467 (23 September 2010), 420–425.

Livadas G., J. Mouchet, J. Gariou, and R. Chastang. "Peut-on envisager l'eradication du paludisme dans la region forestière du Sud Cameroun?," *Rivista di Malariologia*, vol. 37, nos. 4–6 (1958), 229–256.

Livingstone, D. *Narrative of an Expedition to The Zambesi and Its Tributaries* (Torrington, WY: Narrative Press, 2004).

Lodewyck, A. "Note sur la transfusion sanguine chez les nourissons et les enfants," *Recueil de travaux de sciences médicales au Congo belge*, vol. 2 (1944), 157–161.

Loewenson, R. "Structural Adjustment and Health Policy in Africa," *International Journal of Health Services*, vol. 23, no. 4 (1993), 717–730.

Lubbe, A., I. Seibert, I. T. Klimkait, and F. van der Kooy. "Ethnopharmacology in Overdrive: The Remarkable Anti-HIV Activity of *Artemisia annua*," *Journal of Ethnopharmacology*, vol. 141, no. 3 (2012), 854–859.

Mabaso, M. L. H., B. Sharp, and C. Lengeler. "Historical Review of Malarial Control in Southern Africa with Emphasis on the Use of Indoor Residual House-Spraying," *Tropical Medicine and International Health*, vol. 9, no. 8 (2004), 846–856.

MacCormick, C. P., and G. Lwihula. "Failure to Participate in a Malaria Chemosuppression Programme: North Mara, Tanzania," *Journal of Tropical Medicine and Hygiene*, vol. 86, no. 3 (1983), 99–107.

MacCormack, C. P., and R. W. Snow. "Gambian Cultural Preferences in the Use of Insecticide-Impregnated Bed Nets," *Journal of Tropical Medicine and Hygiene*, vol. 89, no. 6 (1986), 295–302.

MacDonald, G. "The Analysis of Malaria Parasite Rates in Infants," *Tropical Diseases Bulletin*, vol. 47, nos. 1–2 (1950), 915–938.

MacDonald, G. "Community Aspects of Immunity to Malaria," *British Medical Bulletin*, vol. 8, no. 1 (1951), 33–36.

MacDonald, G. "The Analysis of Equilibrium in Malaria," *Tropical Diseases Bulletin*, vol. 49, no. 9 (1952), 813–829.

MacDonald, G. "The Epidemiological Basis of Malaria Control," *Bulletin of the World Health Organization*, vol. 15, nos. 3–5 (1956), 613–626.

MacDonald, G. *The Epidemiology and Control of Malaria* (London: Oxford University Press, 1957).

MacDonald, G., and G. Davidson. "Dose and Cycle of Insecticide Applications in the Control of Malaria," *Bulletin of the World Health Organization*, vol. 9, no. 6 (1953), 785–812.

Macfie, J. W. S., and A. Ingram. "Observations on Malaria in the Gold Coast Colony, West Africa," *Annals of Tropical Medicine and Parasitology*, vol. 11 (1918), 1–23.

MacGregor, W., R. Ross, J. M. Young, C. F. Fearnside, G. A. Williamson, G. G. Low, R. W. Boyce, E. Henderson, P. Manson, J. L. Poynder, and J. Cantlie. "A Discussion on Malaria and Its Prevention," *British Medical Journal*, vol. 2, no. 2124 (14 September 1901), 680–690.

Maddison, A. *The World Economy: Historical Statistics* (Paris: OECD [Development Centre of the Organisation for Economic Co-operation and Development, 2003]).

Maegraith, B. *Pathological Processes in Malaria and Blackwater Fever* (Oxford: Blackwell Publications, 1948).

Maegraith, B. G. "Presidential Address on Some Controversial Aspects of Malarial Control," *Journal of the Royal Sanitary Institute*, vol. 70, no. 5 (1950), 445–448.

Makemba, A. M., P. J. Winch, V. M. Makame, G. L. Mehl, Z. Premji, J. N. Minjas, and C. J. Shiff. "Treatment Practices for Degedege, a Locally-Recognized Febrile Illness, and Implications for Strategies to Decrease Mortality from Severe Malaria in Bagamoyo District, Tanzania," *Tropical Medicine and International Health*, vol. 1, no. 3 (1996), 305–313.

Malakooti, M. A., K. Biomndo, and G. D. Shanks. "Reemergence of Epidemic Malaria in the Highlands of Western Kenya," *Emerging Infectious Diseases*, vol. 4, no. 4 (1998), 671–676.

Marchoux, É. "Le paludisme au Sénégal," *Archives de médecine navale*, vol. 68 (1897), 288–308.

Marchoux, É. "Transmission du paludisme par les moustiques," *Annales d'hygiène et de médecine coloniale*, vol. 2 (1899), 22–25.

Marchoux, É. "Tous les alcaloïdes du quinquina possedent la meme action curative sur le paludisme," *Bullétin de la Société de pathologie exotique*, vol. 12 (1919), 307–309.

Marchoux, É. "La fièvre quarte et son mystère," *Revue coloniale de médecine et de chirurgie* (15 October 1930), 213–220.

Marsh, K. "Malaria–A Neglected Disease?," *Parasitology*, vol. 104, issue S1 (1992), s53-s69.

Marsh, K. "Immunology of Malaria," in D. A. Warrell and H. M. Gilles (eds.), *Essential Malariology* (London: Arnold Publishers, 2002), 252–267.

Mason, D. P., and F. E. McKenzie. "Blood Stage Dynamics and Clinical Implications of Mixed *Plasmodium vivax-Plasmodium falciparum* Infections," *American Journal of Tropical Medicine and Hygiene*, vol. 61, no. 3 (1999), 367–374.

Matola, Y. G., and S. A. Magayuka. "Malaria in the Pare Area of Tanzania. V. Malaria 20 years after the End of Residual Insecticide Spraying," *Transactions of the Royal Society of Tropical Medicine and Hygiene*, vol. 75, no. 6 (1981), 811–813.

Matson, A. T. "The History of Malaria in Nandi," *East African Medical Journal*, vol. 3, no. 8 (1957), 431–441.

Mattlet, G. "Quelques considerations sur des cas de fièvre paratyphoïde C et contribution à l'étude des bacilles paratyphoïdes," *Annales de la Société belge de medicine tropicale*, vol. 11, no. 4 (1931), 455–478.

McCombie, S. C. "Treatment Seeking for Malaria: A Review of Recent Research," *Social Science and Medicine*, vol. 43, no. 6 (1996), 933–945.

McGregor, I. A. "Demographic Effects of Malaria with Special Reference to the Stable Malaria of Africa," *West African Medical Journal*, vol. 9, no. 6 (1960), 260–265.

McGregor, I. A. "The Significance of Parasitic Infections in Terms of Clinical Disease: A Personal View," *Parasitology*, vol. 94, supplement S1 (1987), S159–S178.

McGregor, I. A., H. M. Gilles, J. H. Walters, A. H. Davies, and F. A. Pearson. "Effects of Heavy and Repeated Malarial Infections on Gambia Infants and Children," *British Medical Journal*, vol. 2 (22 September 1956), 686–692.

McGregor, I. A., and R. J. M. Wilson. "Precipitating Antibodies and Immunoglobins in P. Falciparum Infections in the Gambia, West Africa," *Transactions of the Royal Society of Tropical Medicine and Hygiene*, vol. 65, no. 2 (1971), 136–151.

McGregor, J., and T. Ranger. "Displacement and Disease: Epidemics and Ideas About Malaria in Matabeleland, Zimbabwe, 1945–1996," *Past and Present*, vol. 167 (2000), 203–237.

McKenzie, A. "The Distribution of Malaria in Dar es-Salaam," *Kenya and East African Medical Journal*, vol. 4 (1927–1928), 164–180.

McNeill, J. R. *Mosquito Empires: Ecology and War in the Greater Caribbean, 1620–1914* (New York: Cambridge University Press, 2010).

Mercier, S., and J. B. Razafindrakoto. "Bilan de trois années de campagnes de désinsectisation domestique à Tananarive," *Bullétin de la Société de pathologie exotique*, vol. 46, no. 3 (1953), 463–473.

Merle, F., and L. Maillot. "Campagnes de désinsectisation contre le paludisme à Brazzaville," *Bullétin de la Société de pathologie exotique*, vol. 48, no. 2 (1955), 242–269.

Michel, R. "Résistance à la pyriméthamine dans la zone antipaludique du Thiès," *Médecine tropicale*, vol. 21, no. 6 (1961), 876–878.

Miller, H. M., and R. N. Singh. "Urbanization during the Postcolonial Days," in James D. Tarver (ed.), *Urbanization in Africa: A Handbook* (Westport, CT: Greenwood Press, 1994), 65–79.

Miller, M. J. "Observations on the Natural History of Malaria in the Semi-Resistant West African," *Transactions of the Royal Society of Tropical Medicine and Hygiene*, vol. 52, no. 2 (1958), 152–168.

Mockenhaupt, F. P., S. Ehrhardt, S. Gellert, R. N. Otchwemah, E. Dietz, S. D. Anemana, and U. Bienzle. "Alpha +-thalassemia Protects African Children from Severe Malaria," *Blood*, vol. 104, no. 7 (2004), 2003–2006.

Möhrle, J., S. Duparc, C. Siethoff, P. L. M. van Giersbergen, J. C. Craft, S. Arbe-Barnes, S. A. Charman, M. Gutierrez, S. Wittlin, and J. L. Vennerstrom. "First-in-Man Safety and Pharmacokinetics of Synthetic Ozonide OZ439 Demonstrates an Improved Exposure Profile Relative to Other Peroxide Antimalarials," *British Journal of Clinical Pharmacology*, vol. 75, no. 2 (2013), 535–548.

Molineaux, L. "Malaria and Mortality: Some Epidemiological Considerations," *Annals of Tropical Medicine and Parasitology*, vol. 91, no. 7 (1977), 811–825.

Molineaux, L., and G. Gramiccia. *The Garki Project: Research on the Epidemiology and Control of Malaria in the Sudan Savanna of West Africa* (Geneva: World Health Organization, 1980).

Morin, H. G. S. "Sur une campagne antipalustre au Cameroun (1953–1954). Premiers résultats de l'enquête épidémiologique," *Rivista de malariologia*, vol. 34, nos. 1–3 (1955), 37–47.

Morin, H. G. S. "Sur une campagne antipalustre au Cameroun (1953–1954). Mesures préventives prises," *Rivista de malariologia*, vol. 34, nos. 4–6 (1955), 191–213.

Mouchet, J., P. Carnevale, M. Coosemans, J. Julvez, S. Manguin, D. Richard-Lenoble, and J. Sircoulon. *Biodiversité du paludisme dans le monde* (Montrouge: Éditions John Libbey Eurotext, 2004).

Mouchet, J., and J. Hamon. "Les problèmes techniques de l'éradication du paludisme en Afrique," *Cahiers O. R. S. T. O. M.*, Série Entomologie Médicale, vol. 33 (1963), 39–48.

Mouchet, J., S. Laventure, S. Blanchy, R. Fioramonti, A. Rakotonjanabelo, P. Rabarison, J. Sircoulon, and J. Roux. "La reconquête des Hautes Terres de Madagascar par le paludisme," *Bullétin de la Société de pathologie exotique*, vol. 90 (1997), 162–168.

Mouchet, J., S. Manguin, J. Sircoulon, S. Laventure, O. Faye, A. W. Onapa, P. Carnevale, J. Julvez, and D. Fontenille. "Evolution of Malaria in Africa for the Past 40 Years: Impact of Climatic and Human Factors," *Journal of the American Mosquito Control Association*, vol. 14, no. 2 (1998), 121–130.

Muela, S. H., J. M. Ribera, and M. Tanner. "Fake Malaria and Hidden Parasites–The Ambiguity of Malaria," *Anthropology & Medicine*, vol. 5, no. 1 (1998), 43–61.

Mueller, I., P. A. Zimmerman, and J. C. Reeder. "*Plasmodium malariae* and *Plasmodium ovale* – the 'Bashful' Malaria Parasites," *Trends in Parasitology*, vol. 23, no. 6 (2007), 278–283.

Muirhead-Thomson, R. C. "Where Do Most Mosquitoes Acquire Their Malarial (*Plasmodium falciparum*) Infection? from Adults or from Children?," *Annals of Tropical Medicine and Parasitology*, vol. 92, no. 8 (1998), 891–893.

Murray, C. J. L., L. C. Rosenfeld, S. S. Lim, K. G. Andrews, K. J. Foreman, D. Haring, N. Fullman, M. Naghavi, R. Lozano, and A. D. Lopez. "Global Malaria Mortality between 1980 and 2010: A Systematic Analysis," *The Lancet*, vol. 379, no. 9814 (4 February 2012), 413–431.

Mutero, C. M., C. Kabutha, V. Kimani, L. Kabuage, G. Gitau, J. Ssennyonga, J. Githure, L. Muthami, A. Kaida, L. Musyoka, E. Kiarie, and M. Oganda. "A Transdisciplinary Perspective on the Links between Malaria and Agroecosystems in Kenya," *Acta Tropica*, vol. 89, no. 2 (2004), 171–186.

Mwai, L., E. Ochong, A. Abdirahman, S. M. Kiara, S. Ward, G. Kokwaro, P. Sasi, K. Marsh, S. Borrmann, M. Mackinnon, and A. Nzila. "Chloroquine Resistance before and after Its Withdrawal in Kenya," *Malaria Journal*, vol. 8 (2009), 1–10. Available online: http://www.malariajournal.com/content/8/1/106

Nájera, J. A. "A Critical Review of the Field Application of a Mathematical Model of Malaria Eradication," *Bulletin of the World Health Organization*, vol. 50, no. 5 (1974), 449–457.

Nájera, J. A. "Malaria Control: Present Situation and Need For Historical Research," *Parassitologia*, vol. 32 (1990), 215–229.

Nájera, J. A. "Tropical Diseases and Socioeconomic Development," *Parassitologia*, vol. 36 (1994), 17–33.

Nájera, J. A. "Malaria Control: Achievements, Problems, and Strategies," *Parassitologia*, vol. 43, nos. 1–2 (2001), 1–89.

Nájera, J. A., G. R. Shidrawi, F. D. Gibson, and J. S. Stafford. "A Large-Scale Field Trial of Malathion as an Insecticide for Antimalarial Work in Southern Uganda," *Bulletin of the World Health Organization*, vol. 36, no. 6 (1967), 913–935.

Nchinda, T. C. "Malaria: A Reemerging Disease in Africa," *Emerging Infectious Diseases*, vol. 4, no. 3 (1998), 398–403.

Ndulu, B. J., and S. A. O'Connell. "Policy Plus: African Growth Performance, 1960–2000," in B. J. Ndulu, S. A. O'Connell, R. H. Bates, P. Collier, and C. C. Soludo (eds.), *The Political Economy of Economic Growth in Africa, 1960–2000*, vol. 1 (New York: Cambridge University Press, 2008), 3–75.

Ndulu, B. J., S. A. O'Connell, R. H. Bates, P. Collier, and C. C. Soludo (eds.). *The Political Economy of Economic Growth in Africa, 1960–2000*, vol. 1 (New York: Cambridge University Press, 2008).

Newman, P. *Malaria Eradication and Population Growth with Special Reference to Ceylon and British Guiana* (Ann Arbor: University of Michigan Press, 1965).

Nnochiri, E. *Parasitic Disease and Urbanization in a Developing Community* (London: Oxford University Press, 1968).

Nogver, A., W. Wernsdorfer, R. Kovznetsov, and J. Hempel. "The Malaria Situation in 1976," *World Health Organization Chronicle*, vol. 32, no. 1 (1978), 9–17.

Nuwaha, F., J. Babirye, and N. Ayiga. "Why the Increase in under-Five Mortality in Uganda from 1995 to 2000? A Retrospective Analysis," *BMC Public Health*, vol. 11 (2011), 725. Available online: http://www.biomedcentral.com/1471-2458/11/725

Ogutu, R. O., A. J. Oloo, W. S. Ekissa, I. O. Genga, N. Mulaya, and J. I. Githure. "The Effect of Participatory School Health Programme on the Control of Malaria," *East African Medical Journal*, vol. 69, no. 6 (1992), 298–302.

Okumu, F. O., N. J. Govella, S. J. Moore, N. Chitnis, and G. F. Killeen. "Potential Benefits, Limitations and Target Product-Profiles of Odor-Baited Mosquito Traps for Malaria Control in Africa," *PLOS ONE*, vol. 5, no. 7 (2010), 1–18.

Oloo, A. J., J. M. Vulule, and D. K. Koech, "Some Emerging Issues on the Malaria Problem in Kenya," *East African Medical Journal*, vol. 73, no. 1 (1996), 50–53.

Ombongi, K., and M. Rutten. "Dashed Hopes and Missed Opportunities: Malaria Control Policies in Kenya (1896–2009)," in M. Dekker and R. van Dijk (eds.), *Markets of Well-Being: Navigating Health and Healing in Africa* (Leiden: Brill, 2010), 109–143.

Ombongi, K. S., M. Dobson, M. Malowany, and R. S. Snow. "The East African Medical Journal: Its History and Contribution to Regional Malaria Research during the Last 75 Years," *East African Medical Journal*, 75, 1998, s10–19.

Ongore, D., F. Kamunvi, R. Knight, and A. Minawa. "Malaria and the Mosquito Vector–A Study of Knowledge, Attitudes, and Practices [KAP] of a Rural Community," *East African Medical Journal*, vol. 66, no. 2 (1989), 79–90.

Onori, E. "The Problem of *Plasmodium falciparum* Drug Resistance in Africa South of the Sahara," *Bulletin of the World Health Organization*, vol. 62, supplement (1984), 55–62.

Onori, E. "Epidemiological Considerations on the Occurrence and Geographical Distribution of *Plasmodium falciparum* Resistance to Antimalarials in Africa," *La Medicina Tropicale Nella Cooperazione Allo Sviluppo*, vol. 3, no. 1 (1987), 23–40.

Onori, E., B. Grab, P. Ambroise-Thomas, and J. Thelu. "Incipient Status of *Plasmodium falciparum* to Chloroquine among a Semi-Immune Population of the United Republic of Tanzania," *Bulletin of the World Health Organization*, vol. 60, no. 6 (1982), 899–906.

Otoo, L. N., R. W. Snow, A. Menon, P. Byass, and B. M. Greenwood. "Immunity to Malaria in Young Gambian Children after a Two-Year Period of Chemoprophylaxis," *Transactions of the Royal Society of Tropical Medicine and Hygiene*, vol. 82, no. 1 (1988), 59–65.

Paaijmans, K. P., S. Blanford, B. H. K. Chan, and M. B. Thomas. "Warmer Temperatures Reduce the Vectorial Capacity of Malaria Mosquitoes," *Biology Letters*, vol. 8, no. 3 (2012), 465–468.

Packard, R. "'Malaria Blocks Development' Revisited: The Role of Disease in the History of Agricultural Development in the Eastern and Northern Transvaal Lowveld, 1890–1960," *Journal of Southern African Studies*, vol. 27, no. 3 (2001), 591–612.

Packard, R. *The Making of a Tropical Disease: A Short History of Malaria* (Baltimore: Johns Hopkins University Press, 2007).

Packard, R. M. "Maize, Cattle, and Mosquitoes: The Political Economy of Malaria Epidemics in Colonial Swaziland," *Journal of African History*, vol. 25, no. 2 (1984), 189–212.

Packard, R. M. "Agricultural Development, Labor Migration, and the Resurgence of Malaria in Swaziland," *Social Science and Medicine*, vol. 22, no. 8 (1986), 861–867.

Packard, R. M. "'Roll Back Malaria, Roll in Development?': Reassessing the Economic Burden of Malaria," *Population and Development Review*, vol. 35, no. 1 (2009), 53–87.

Packard, R. M., and P. Gadelha. "A Land Filled with Mosquitoes: Fred L. Soper, the Rockefeller Foundation, and the *Anopheles gambiae* Invasion of Brazil," *Parassitologia*, vol. 36 (1994), 197–213.

Padonou, G. G., M. Sezonlin, R. Ossé, N. Aizoun, F. Oké-Agbo, O. Oussou, G. Gbédjissi, and M. Akogbéto. "Impact of Three Years of Large Scale Indoor Residual Spraying (IRS) and Insecticide Treated Nets (ITNs) Interventions on Insecticide Resistance in *Anopheles gambiae s. l.* in Benin," *Parasites and Vectors*, vol. 5, issue, 1, no. 72 (2012). Available online: http://www.Parasitesandvectors.Com/Content/Pdf/1756-3305-5-72.Pdf

Pakenham, T. *The Scramble for Africa: White Man's Conquest of the Dark Continent from 1876–1912* (New York: Random House, 1991).

Pålsson, K., and T. G. T. Jaenson. "Plant Products Used as Mosquito Repellents in Guinea Bissau, West Africa," *Acta Tropica*, vol. 72, no. 1 (1999), 39–52.

Pan-African Health Conference. "Malaria under African Conditions," *Quarterly Bulletin of the Health Organization of the League of Nations*, vol. 5 (1936), 110–137.

Parent, G., J. Vercruysse, P. Gazin, J. Roffi, R. Slavov, and M. Blanchot. "Paludisme, anémie et état nutritionnel: Étude longitudinale et interactions en zone sahélienne (Sénégal)," *Bullétin de la Société de pathologie exotique*, vol. 80, no. 3 (1987), 546–560.

Park Ross, G. A. "Insecticide as a Major Measure in the Control of Malaria, Being an Account of the Methods and Organisation Put in Force in Natal and Zululand during the Past Six Years," *Quarterly Bulletin of the Health Organisation of the League of Nations*, vol. 5 (1936), 114–133.

Parmakelis, A., M. A. Russello, A. Caccone, C. B. Marcondes, J. Costa, O. P. Forattini, M. A. M. Sallum, R. C. Wilkinson, and J. R. Powell. "Short Report: Historical Analysis of a Near Disaster: *Anopheles gambiae* in Brazil," *American Journal of Tropical Medicine and Hygiene*, vol. 78, no. 1 (2008), 176–178.

Paterson, A. R. "General Antimalaria Measures: The Lesson of the History of Malaria in the United States of America," *Kenya and East African Medical Journal*, vol. 7, no. 7 (1930), 180–189.

Patterson, G. *The Mosquito Crusades: A History of the American Anti-Mosquito Movement from the Reed Commission to the First Earth Day* (New Brunswick, NJ: Rutgers University Press, 2009).

Patterson, K. D. *Infectious Diseases in Twentieth Century Africa: A Bibliography of Their Distribution and Consequences* (Waltham, MA: Crossroads Press, 1979).

Patterson, K. D. *Health in Colonial Ghana: Disease, Medicine, and Socio-Economic Change, 1900–1955* (Waltham, MA: Crossroads Press, 1981).

Payne, D., B. Grah, R. E. Fontaine, and J. H. G. Hempel. "Impact of Control Measures on Malaria Transmission and General Mortality," *Bulletin of the World Health Organization*, vol. 54, no. 4 (1976), 369–377.

Peaston, H., and E. A. Renner. "Report on an Examination of the Spleen- and Parasite-Rates in School Children in Freetown, Sierra, Leone," *Annals of Tropical Medicine and Parasitology*, vol. 33 (1939), 49–59.

Pehrson, P. O., A. Björkman, J. Brohult, L. Jorfeldt, P. Lundbergh, L. Rombo, M. Willcox, and E. Bengtsson. "Is the Working Capacity of Liberian Industrial Workers Increased by Regular Malaria Prophylaxis?," *Annals of Tropical Medicine and Parasitology*, vol. 78, no. 5 (1984), 453–458.

Peters, W. *Malaria Eradication in Tropical Africa* (Port Moresby, Territory of Papua and New Guinea: Department of Public Health, Malaria Section, 1960).

Phoofolo, P. "Epidemics and Revolutions: The Rinderpest Epidemic in Late Nineteenth Century Southern Africa," *Past and Present*, vol. 138, no. 1 (1993), 112–143.

Picard, J., M. Aikins, P. L. Alonso, J. M. R. Armstrong Schellenberg, B. M. Greenwood, and A. Mills. "A Malaria Control Trial Using Insecticide-Treated Bed Nets and Targeted Chemoprophylaxis in a Rural Area of The Gambia, West Africa. 8. Cost-Effectiveness of Bed Net Impregnation Alone or Combined with Chemoprophylaxis in Preventing Mortality and Morbidity from Malaria in Gambian Children," *Transactions of the Royal Society of Tropical Medicine and Hygiene*, vol. 87, supplement 2 (1993), 53–57.

Pison, G., J.-F. Trape, M. Lefebvre, and C. Enel. "Rapid Decline in Child Mortality in a Rural Area of Senegal," *International Journal of Epidemiology*, vol. 22, no. 1 (1993), 72–80.

Pringle, G. "The Effect of Social Factors in Reducing the Intensity of Malaria Transmission in Coastal East Africa," *Transactions of the Royal Society of Tropical Medicine and Hygiene*, vol. 60, no. 4 (1966), 549–553.

Pringle, G., C. C. Draper, and D. F. Clyde. "A New Approach to the Measurement of Residual Transmission in a Malaria Control Scheme in East Africa," *Transactions of the Royal Society of Tropical Medicine and Hygiene*, vol. 54, no. 5 (1960), 434–438.

Pringle, W., and S. Avery-Jones. "Observation on the Early Course of Untreated Falciparum Malaria in Semi-Immune African Children Following a Short Period of Protection," *Bulletin of the World Health Organization*, vol. 34, no. 2 (1966), 269–272.

Projet Santé Pour Tous. "Le paludisme dans la population de Kinshasa: Perception du problème, moyens d'action, evaluation," *Annales de la Société belge de médicine tropicale*, vol. 65, supplement 2 (1985), 215–222.

Prothero, R. M. "Population Movements and Problems of Malaria Eradication in Africa," *Bulletin of the World Health Organization*, vol. 24, nos. 4–5 (1961), 405–425.

Prothero, R. M. *Migrants and Malaria* (London: Longman, 1965).

Prugnolle, F., V. Rougeron, P. Becquart, A. Berry, B. Makanga, N. Rahola, C. Arnathau, B. Ngoubangoye, S. Menard, E. Willaume, F. J. Ayala, D. Fontenille, B. Ollomo, P. Durand, C. Paupy, and F. Renaud, "Diversity, Host Switching and Evolution of *Plasmodium vivax* Infecting Great Apes," *Proceedings of the National Academy of Sciences*, vol. 110, no. 20 (2013), 8123–8128.

Quenum, A. "Les vicissitudes des programmes d'éradication du paludisme en Afrique," *Médicine d'Afrique Noire*, vol. 14 (1963), 287–291.

Ranson, H., R. N'Guessan, J. Lines, N. Moiroux, Z. Nkuni, and V. Corbel. "Pyrethroid Resistance in African Anopheline Mosquitoes: What Are the Implications for Malaria Control?," *Trends in Parasitology*, vol. 27, no. 2 (2011), 91–98.

Restif, O. "Evolutionary Epidemiology 20 Years On: Challenges and Prospects," *Infection, Genetics and Evolution*, vol. 9, no. 1 (2009), 108–123.

Ribeiro, L. "Notas Sôbre Aspectos Nosofráficos das Endemias de Angola (I Parte)," *Separata* [supplement] of the *Boletim Sanitáro* (1942), 5–12.

Riehle, M. M., W. M. Guelbeogo, A. Gneme, K. Eiglmeier, I. Holm, E. Bischoff, T. Garnier, G. M. Snyder, X. Li, K. Markianos, N'F. Sagnon, and K. D. Vernick. "A Cryptic Subgroup of *Anopheles gambiae* Is Highly Susceptible to Human Malaria Parasites," *Science*, vol. 331 (4 February 2011), 596–598.

Rimbaut, G., and M. Mathis. "Utilisation des "Poissons Millions" pour la lutte biologique contre les larves d'anophèles à Dakar," *Bullétin de la Société de pathologie exotique*, vol. 28, no. 7 (1935), 10–18.

Rivero, A., J. Vézilier, M. Weill, A. F. Read, and S. Gandon. "Insecticide Control of Vector-Borne Diseases: When Is Insecticide Resistance a Problem?," *PLOS Pathogens*, vol. 6, no. 8 (2010), 1–9.

Robert, V., K. Macintyre, J. Keating, J.-F. Trape, J.-B. Duchemin, M. Warren, and J. C. Beier. "Malaria Transmission in Urban Sub-Saharan Africa," *American Journal of Tropical Medicine and Hygiene*, vol. 68, no. 2 (2003), 169–176.

Robert, V., J. -F. Molez, and C. Becker. "L'évolution de la recherche et de la lutte contre le paludisme en Afrique de l'Ouest au XXème siècle," in C. Becker, S. Mbaye, and I. Thioub (eds.), *A. O. F.: Réalités et heritages. Sociétés ouest-africaines et ordre colonial, 1895–1960*, vol. 2 (Dakar: Direction des Archives Nationales du Sénégal, 1997), 1175–1186.

Roberts, D., and R. Tren. *The Excellent Powder: DDT's Political and Scientific History* (Indianapolis: Dog Ear Publishing, 2010).

Roberts, J. M. D. "Pyrimethamine (Daraprim) in the Control of Epidemic Malaria," *Journal of Tropical Medicine and Hygiene*, vol. 59, no. 9 (1956), 201–208.

Roberts, J. M. D. "The Control of Epidemic Malaria in the Highlands of Western Kenya. Part I. before the Campaign," *Journal of Tropical Medicine and Hygiene*, vol. 67 (July 1964), 161–168; *Journal of Tropical Medicine and Hygiene*, "Part II. The Campaign," vol. 67 (August, 1964), 191–199; and "Part III. after the Campaign," *Journal of Tropical Medicine and Hygiene*, vol. 67 (September 1964), 230–237.

Rodhain, J. "La prophylaxie antimalarienne dans les regions tropicales envisagée à la lumière des récents progrès thérapeutiques, *Bullétin de l'Institut Royale Colonial Belge*, vol. 4 (1933), 649–667.

Rodhain, J. "Compte rendu des Travaux des Commissions chargées d'étudier l'organisation de la lutte contre le paludisme au Congo Belge et au Ruandi-Urundi," *Bullétin de l'Institut Royal Colonial Belge*, vol. 22, no. 3 (1951), 3–53.

Rogier, C., T. Fusaï, B. Pradines, and J.-F. Trape. "Comment évaluer la morbidité attributable au paludisme en zone d'endémie?," *Revue d'épidémiologie et de santé publique*, vol. 53, no. 3 (2005), 299–309.

Rønn, A. M., H. A. Msangeni, J. Mhina, W. H. Wernsdorfer, and I. C. Bygbjerg. "High Level of Resistance of *Plasmodium falciparum* to Sulfadoxine-Pyrimethamine in Children in Tanzania," *Transactions of the Royal Society of Tropical Medicine and Hygiene*, vol. 90, no. 2 (1996), 179–181.

Ronsse, C. S. "Anémies malariennes des enfants et transfusions sanguines; avec observations sur les groupes sanguins des Bakongo," *Mémoires de l'Institut Royal Colonial Belge, Section des Sciences Naturelles et Médicales*, vol. 20 (1952), 1–64.

Ross, R. *Report of the Malaria Expedition to Sierra Leone (1899)*. Memoir I (London: University of Liverpool Press, 1899).

Ross, R. *First Progress Report of the Campaign against Mosquitoes in Sierra Leone (1901)*. Memoir V, Part I (London: University Press of Liverpool, 1901).

Rowe, A. K., A. Y. Rowe, R. W. Snow, E. L. Korenromp, J. R. M. Armstrong Schellenberg, C. Stein, B. L. Nahlen, J. Bryce, R. E. Black, and R. W. Steketee. "The Burden of Malaria Mortality among African Children in the Year 2000," *International Journal of Epidemiology*, vol. 35, no. 3 (2006), 691–704.

The RTS, S Clinical Trials Partnership. "First Results of Phase 3 Trial of RTS, S/AS01 Malaria Vaccine in African Children," *New England Journal of Medicine*, vol. 365 (2011), 1863–75.

The RTS, S Clinical Trials Partnership. "A Phase 3 Trial of RTS, S/AS01 Malaria Vaccine in African Children," *New England Journal of Medicine*, vol. 367 (2012), 2284–2295.

Sabatinelli, G. et al. "Prevalence du paludisme à Ouagadougou et dans le milieu rural limitrophe en période de transmission maximale," *Parassitologia*, vol. 28, no. 1 (1986), 17–31.

Sabben-Clare, E. E., D. J. Bradley, and K. Kirkwood (eds.), *Health in Tropical Africa during the Colonial Period* (Oxford: Clarendon Press, 1980).

Sachs, J. and P. Malaney, "The Economic and Social Burden of Malaria," *Nature*, vol. 415 (7 February 2002), 680–685.

Sahn, D., and R. Bernier. "Have Structural Adjustments Led to Health Sector Reform in Africa?," *Health Policy*, vol. 32, nos. 1–3 (1995), 193–214.

Salako, L. A. "Quinine and Malaria: The African Experience," *Acta Leidensia*, vol. 55 (1987), 167–180.

Sankale, M., B. Diop, and I. Gueye. "Enquête d'opinion sur le paludisme en milieu rural au Sénégal," *Médecine d'Afrique Noire*, no. 6 (June 1967), 271–280.

Sanner, L., and A. Masseguin. "Le Service d'Hygiène Mobile et son oeuvre," *Bullétin Médical de l'Afrique Occidentale Française*, special issue (January 1954), 9–59.

Schneider, J., J. Languillon, and A. Delas. "Association choloroquine-pyriméthamine dans la chimioprophylaxie du paludisme: Résultats après 22 mois de traitement," *Bullétin de la Société de pathologie exotique*, vol. 51 (1958), 316–319.

Schneider, W. H. *A History of Blood Transfusion in Sub-Saharan Africa* (Athens: Ohio University Press, 2013).

Schram, R. *A History of the Nigerian Health Services* (Ibadan: Ibadan University Press, 1971).

Schüffner, W. A. P. "Two Subjects Relating to the Epidemiology of Malaria," *Journal of the Malaria Institute of India*, vol. 1, no. 3 (1938), 221–256.

Schüffner, W. A. P., N. H. Swellengrebel, S. Anneke, and B. de Meillon, "Vergleichende Untersuchungen über Malariaimmunität in Niederlandisch-Indien und Südafrika," *Zentralblatt für Bakteriologie*, 125 Band, Heft 1/2, July 1932.

Schultz, L. J., R. W. Steketee, A. Macheso, P. Kazembe, L. Chitsulo, and J. J. Wirima. "The Efficacy of Antimalarial Regimens Containing Sulfadoxine-Pyrimethamine and/or Chloroquine in Preventing Peripheral and Placental *Plasmodium falciparum* Infection among Pregnant Women in Malawi," *American Journal of Tropical Medicine and Hygiene*, vol. 51, no. 5 (1994), 515–522.

Schumaker, L. "The Mosquito Taken at the Beerhall," in P. W. Geissler and C. Molyneux (eds.), *Evidence, Ethos, and Experiment: The Anthropology and History of Medical Research in Africa* (New York: Berghahn Books, 2011), 403–427.

Schwalbach, J. F. L., and M. C. R. Dela Maza. *A Malária em Moçambique [1937–1973]* (n. p.: Instituto Nacional de Saude, n. d. [circa 1974]).

Schwetz, J. "Le mystère de la fièvre quarte et tierce bénigne en Afrique Équatoriale et Centrale," *Bullétin de pathologie exotique*, vol. 25 (1932), 1062–1074.

Schwetz, J. "Quelques considérations et réflexions sur l'immunité malarienne," *Rivista di Malariologia*, vol. 13, no. 5 (1934), 669–678.

Schwetz, J. "Considerations sur la future lutte anti-anophélo-paludéenne au moyen du D. D. T. au Congo Belge, resp. en Afrique centrale," *Annales de la Société belge de médecine tropicale*, vol. 28 (1948), 1–33.

Scott, J. C. *Seeing Like a State: How Certain Schemes to Improve the Human Condition Have Failed* (New Haven, CT: Yale University Press, 1999).

Scott, R. R. "Public Health Services in Dar es-Salaam in the Twenties," *East African Medical Journal*, vol. 40, no. 7 (1963), 339–353.

Shaffer, N., K. Hedberg, F. Davachi, B. Lyamba, J. G. Breman, O. Samu Masisa, F. Behets, A. Hightower, and P. Nguyen-Dinh. "Trends and Risk Factors for HIV-1 Seropositivity among Outpatient Children, Kinshasa, Zaire," *AIDS*, vol. 4, no. 12 (1990): 1231–1236.

Sherman, I. W. *The Elusive Malaria Vaccine: Miracle or Mirage?* (Washington, DC: American Society for Microbiology, 2009).

Sherman, I. W. *Magic Bullets to Conquer Malaria: From Quinine to Qinghaosu* (Washington, DC: American Society for Microbiology, 2011).

Shore, W. H. *The Imaginations of Unreasonable Men: Inspiration, Vision, and Purpose in the Quest to End Malaria* (New York: Public Affairs, 2010).

Shousha, A. T. "The Eradication of *Anopheles gambiae* from Upper Egypt, 1942–1945," *Bulletin of the World Health Organization*, vol. 1, no. 2 (1948), 309–352.

Sissoko, M. S., A. Dicko, O. J. T. Briët, M. Sissoko, I. Sagara, H. D. Keita, M. Sogoba, C. Rogier, Y. T. Touré, and O. K. Doumbo. "Malaria Incidence in Relation to Rice Cultivation in the Irrigated Sahel of Mali," *Acta Tropica*, vol. 89, no. 2 (2004), 161–170.

Slater, L. B. *War and Disease: Biomedical Research on Malaria in the Twentieth Century* (New Brunswick, NJ: Rutgers University Press, 2009).

Slutsker, L., J. G. Bremen, and C. C. Campbell. "Strategies for Control of Malaria in Africa," *The Lancet* (30 July 1988), 283.

Small, J., S. J. Goetz, and S. I. Hay. "Climatic Suitability for Malaria Transmission in Africa, 1911–1995," *Proceedings of the National Academy of Sciences*, vol. 100, no. 26 (2003), 15341–15345.

Smith, A., C. F. Hansford, and J. F. Thomson. "Malaria Along the Southernmost Fringe of Its Distribution in Africa: Epidemiology and Control," *Bulletin of the World Health Organization*, vol. 55, no. 1 (1977), 95–103.

Smith, A., C. F. Hansford, and J. F. Thomson. "Malaria Control: Epidemiological Research in Southern Africa," *WHO Chronicle*, vol. 31 (1977), 105–107.

Snow, R. W., A. K. Bradley, R. Hayes, P. Byass, and B. M. Greenwood. "Does Woodsmoke Protect against Malaria?," *Annals of Tropical Medicine and Parasitology*, vol. 81, no. 4 (1987), 449–451.

Snow, R. W., S. W. Lindsay, R. J. Hayes, and B. W. Greenwood. "Permethrin-Treated Bed Nets (Mosquito Nets) Prevent Malaria in Gambian Children," *Transactions of the Royal Society of Tropical Medicine and Hygiene*, vol. 82, no. 6 (1988), 838–842.

Snow, R. W., and K. Marsh. "Will Reducing *Plasmodium falciparum* Transmission Alter Malaria Mortality among African Children," *Parasitology Today*, vol. 11, no. 5 (1995), 188–190.

Snow, R. W., and K. Marsh. "New Insights Into the Epidemiology of Malaria Relevant for Disease Control," *British Medical Bulletin*, vol. 54, no. 2 (1998), 293–309.

Snow, R. W., and K. Marsh. "The Epidemiology of Clinical Malaria among African Children," *Bullétin de l'Institut Pasteur*, vol. 96, no. 1 (1998), 15–23.

Snow, R. W., and K. Marsh, "The Consequences of Reducing Transmission of *Plasmodium falciparum* in Africa," *Advances in Parasitology*, vol. 52 (2002), 235–264.

Snow, R. W., N. Peshu, D. Forster, H. Mwenesi, and K. Marsh. "The Role of Shops in the Treatment and Prevention of Childhood Malaria on the Coast of Kenya,"

Transactions of the Royal Society of Tropical Medicine and Hygiene, vol. 86, no. 3 (1992), 237–239.

Snow, R. W., and J. A. Omumbo. "Malaria," in D. T. Jamison, R. G. Feachem, M. W. Makgoba, E. R. Bos, F. K. Baingana, K. J. Hofman, and K. O. Rogo (eds.), *Disease and Mortality in Sub-Saharan Africa* (Washington, DC: The World Bank, 2006), 195–214.

Snow, R. W., J. A. Omumbo, B. Lowe, C. S. Molyneux, J. O. Obiero, A. Palmer, M. W. Weber, M. Pinder, B. Nahlen, C. Obonyo, C. Newbold, S. Gupta, and K. Marsh. "Relation between Severe Malaria Morbidity in Children and Level of *Plasmodium falciparum* Transmission in Africa," *The Lancet*, vol. 349 (7 June 1997), 1650–1654.

Snow, R. W., J.-F. Trape, and K. Marsh, "The Past, Present, and Future of Childhood Malaria Mortality in Africa," *Trends in Parasitology*, vol. 17, no. 2 (2001), 593–597.

Snowden, F. M. *The Conquest of Malaria: Italy, 1900–1962* (New Haven, CT: Yale University Press, 2006).

Soeiro, A. "A Malária em Moçambique, Com Espeical Referência à Campanha Antimalárica Numa Região Predominantemente Urbana (Lourenço Marques) e Uma Região Predominantemente Rural (Vale do Limpopo)," *Anais do Instituto de Medecina Tropical*, vol. 13, no. 4 (1956), 615–634.

Soeiro, A., M. Pereira, and A. Pereira. "A Luta Anti-Malárica em Lourenço Marques," *Anais do Instituto de Medecina Tropical*, vol. 13, no. 4 (1956), 635–669.

Somandjinga, M., M. Lluberas, and W. R. Jobin, "Difficulties in Organizing First Indoor Spray Programme against Malaria under the President's Malaria Initiative," *Bulletin of the World Health Organization*, vol. 87, no. 11 (2009), 871–874.

Soper, F. L. "Species Sanitation as Applied to the Eradication of (A) an Invading or (B) an Indigenous Species," *Proceedings of the Fourth International Congress on Tropical Medicine and Malaria*, vol. 1 (Washington, DC: US Government Printing Office, 1948), 850–857.

Soper, F. L. "The Epidemiology of a Disappearing Disease: Malaria," *American Journal of Tropical Medicine and Hygiene*, vol. 9, no. 1 (1960), 357–366.

Soper, F. L. *Ventures in World Health. The Memoirs of Fred Lowe Soper*. Edited by John Duffy (Washington, DC: Pan American Health Organization, 1977).

Soper, F. L., and D. B. Wilson, *Anopheles gambiae in Brazil, 1930 to 1940* (New York: The Rockefeller Foundation, 1943).

Spencer, H. C., D. C. O. Kaseje, W. E. Collins, M. G. Shehata, A. Turner, P. S. Stanfill, A. Y. Huong, J. M. Roberts, M. Villinski, and D. K. Koech. "Community-Based Malaria Control in Saradidi, Kenya: Description of the Programme and Impact on Parasitaemia Rates and Antimalarial Antibodies," *Annals of Tropical Medicine and Parasitology*, vol. 81, supplement 1 (1987), 13–23.

Spielman, A., U. Kitron, and R. J. Pollack. "Time Limitation and the Role of Research in the Worldwide Attempt to Eradicate Malaria," *Journal of Medical Entomology*, vol. 30, no. 1 (1993), 6–19.

Spinage, C. A. *Cattle Disease: A History* (New York: Springer Publishing, 2003).

Spitzer, L. "The Mosquito and Segregation in Sierra Leone," *Canadian Journal of African Studies*, vol. 2, no. 1 (1968), 49–61.

Stafford Smith, D. M. "Mosquito Records from the Republic of Niger, with reference to the Construction of the New 'Trans-Sahara Highway,'" *Journal of Tropical Medicine and Hygiene*, vol. 84 (1981), 95–100.

Stanisic, D. I., I. Mueller, I. Betuela, P. Siba, and L. Schofield. "Robert Koch Redux: Malaria Immunology in Papua New Guinea," *Parasite Immunology*, vol. 32, no. 8 (2010), 623–632.

Stapleton, D. H. "The Dawn of DDT and Its Experimental Use by the Rockefeller Foundation in Mexico, 1943–1952," *Parassitologia*, vol. 40 (1998), 149–158.

Stearns, J. K. *Dancing in the Glory of Monsters: The Collapse of the Congo and the Great War of Africa* (New York: Public Affairs, 2011).

Stein, P., N. P. Gora, and B. M. Macheka. "Self-Medication with Chloroquine for Malaria Prophylaxis in Urban and Rural Zimbabweans," *Tropical and Geographical Medicine*, vol. 40, no. 3 (1988), 264–268.

Stephens, J. W. W., and S. R. Christophers. "The Malarial Infection of Native Children," in *Reports to the Malaria Committee of the Royal Society*, third series (London: Harrison and Sons, 1900), 4–14.

Stephens, J. W. W., and S. R. Christophers, "On the Destruction of *Anopheles* in Lagos," in *Reports to the Malarial Committee of the Royal Society*, third series (London: Harrison and Sons, 1900), 14–20.

Stephens, J. W. W., and S. R. Christophers, "Note on Malarial Fever Contracted on Railways (under Construction)," in *Reports to the Malarial Committee of the Royal Society*, third series (London: Harrison and Sons, 1900), 20–21.

Stephens, J. W. W., and S. R. Christophers. "The Proposed Site for European Residences in the Freetown Hill," in *Reports to the Malaria Committee of the Royal Society*, fifth series (London, 1901), 1–5.

Storey, J. "A Review of Malaria Work in Sierra Leone 1900 to 1964," *West African Medical Journal*, vol. 21, no. 3 (1972), 57–68.

Strangeways-Dixon, D. "Paludrine (Proguanil) as a Malarial Prophylactic Amongst African Labour in Kenya," *East African Medical Journal*, vol. 27 (1950), 127–130.

Subapriya, R., and S. Nagini, "Medical Properties of Neem Leaves: A Review," *Current Medical Chemistry–Anti-Cancer Agents*, vol. 5, no. 2 (2005), 149–156.

Swellengrebel, N. H. "Réflexions à propos de la Conférence sur le paludisme de Kampala (1950)," *Annales de la Société belge de médecine tropicale*, vol. 31 (1950), 111–119.

Swellengrebel, N. H. "The Parasite-Host Relationship in Malaria," *Annals of Tropical Medicine and Parasitology*, vol. 44, no. 1 (1950), 84–92.

Swellengrebel, N. H. "Parasitology: A Chapter of Ecology," *Documenta de medicina geographica et tropica*, vol. 8, no. 3 (1956), 274–280.

Symes, C. B. "Notes on Anophelines and Malaria in Kenya," *The Kenya and East African Medical Journal*, vol. 5, no. 5 (1928), 138–183.

Symes, C. B. "Report on Anophelines and Malaria in the Trans-Nzoia District," *Kenya and East African Medical Journal*, vol. 8, no. 3 (1931), 64–77 and vol. 8, no. 4 (1931), 108–121.

Symes, C. B. "Malaria in Nairobi," *East African Medical Journal*, vol. 17 (1940), 291–307 and vol. 17 (1941), 414–430.

Symes, C. B. "Initial Experiments in the Use of DDT against Mosquitoes in British Guiana," *Bulletin of Entomological Research*, vol. 37, no. 3 (1947), 399–430.

Symes, C. B. "Some Recent Progress in the Study of Insecticides and Their Application for the Control of Vectors of Disease," *Journal of the Royal Sanitary Institute*, vol. 72, no. 5 (1952), 498–512.

Talisuna, A. O., P. Bloland, and U. D'Alessandro. "History, Dynamics, and Public Health Importance of Malaria Parasite Resistance," *Clinical Microbiology Reviews*, vol. 17, no. 1 (2004), 235–254.

Taylor, M. L. "Sanitary Work in West Africa," *British Medical Journal*, vol. 2, no. 2177 (20 September 1902), 852–853.

Taylor, M. L. *Second Progress Report of the Campaign against Mosquitoes in Sierra Leone*. Memoir V, Part II (London: University Press of Liverpool, 1902).

Taylor, M. L. *Report on the Sanitary Conditions of Cape Coast Town (1902)*. Memoir VIII (London: University Press of Liverpool, 1902).

Taylor, P., and S. L. Mutambu. "A Review of the Malaria Situation in Zimbabwe with Special Reference to the Period 1972–1981," *Transactions of the Royal Society of Tropical Medicine and Hygiene*, vol. 80, no. 1 (1986), 12–19.

Taylor, P., and S. L. Mutambu. "Compliance with Malaria Chemoprophylaxis Programmes in Zimbabwe," *Acta Tropica*, vol. 44, no. 4 (1987), 423–431.

Thiam, S., R. Shoo, and J. Carter. "Are Insecticide Treated Bednets Failing?," *Lancet Infectious Diseases*, vol. 12, no. 7 (2012), 512–514.

Thomson, J. G. "Endemic and Epidemic Malaria in Southern Rhodesia," *Proceedings of the Royal Society of Medicine* vol. 22, no. 8 (26 April 1929), 1052–1058.

Thomson, J. G. "Immunity in Malaria," *Transactions of the Royal Society of Tropical Medicine and Hygiene*, vol. 26, no. 6 (1933), 483–498.

Thomson, J. G. "Malaria in Nyasaland," *Proceedings of the Royal Society of Medicine*, vol. 28, no. 4 (1934), 391–404.

Thomson, M., S. Connor, S. Bennett, U. D'Allesandro, P. Milligan, M. Aikins, P. Langerock, M. Jawara, and B. Greenwood. "Geographical Perspectives on Bednet Use and Malaria Transmission in the Gambia, West Africa," *Social Science and Medicine*, vol. 43, no. 1 (1996), 101–112.

Thuilliez, J., M. S. Sissoko, O. B. Toure, P. Kamate, J.-C. Berthélmy, and O. K. Doumbo. "Malaria and Primary Education in Mali: A Longitudinal Study in the Village of Donéguébougou," *Social Science and Medicine*, vol. 71, no. 2 (2010), 324–334.

Tikasingh, E., C. Edwards, P. J. S. Hamilton, L. M. Commissiong, and C. C. Draper. "A Malaria Outbreak Due to *Plasmodium malariae* on the Island of Grenada," *American Journal of Tropical Medicine and Hygiene*, vol. 29, no. 5 (1980), 715–719.

Tognotti, E. "Program to Eradicate Malaria in Sardinia, 1946–1950," *Emerging Infectious Diseases*, vol. 15, no. 9 (2009), 1460–1466.

Trape, J.-F. "Malaria and Urbanization in Central Africa: The Example of Brazzaville. Part I: Description of the Town and Review of Previous Surveys," *Transactions of the Royal Society for Tropical Medicine and Hygiene*, vol. 81, supplement 2 (1987), 1–9.

Trape, J.-F. "The Public Health Impact of Chloroquine Resistance in Africa," *American Journal of Tropical Medicine and Hygiene*, vol. 64, nos. 1–2 (2001), 12–17.

Trape, J.-F., G. Pison, M.-P. Preziosi, C. Enel, A. Desgrées du Loû, V. Delaunay, B. Samb, E. Lagarde, J.-F. Molez, and F. Simondon. "Impact of Chloroquine Resistance on Malaria Mortality," *Compte Rendus de l'Académie des Sciences*, vol. 321, no. 8 (1998), 689–697.

Trape, J.-F., M. C. Quinet, S. Nzingoula, P. Senga, F. Tchichelle, B. Carme, D. Candito, H. Mayanda, and A. Zoulani. "Malaria and Urbanization in Central Africa: The Example of Brazzaville. Part V: Pernicious Attacks and Mortality," *Transactions of the Royal Society for Tropical Medicine and Hygiene*, vol. 81, supplement 2 (1987), 34–42.

Trape, J.-F., and C. Rogier. "Combating Malaria Morbidity and Mortality by Reducing Transmission," *Parasitology Today*, vol. 12, no. 6 (1996), 236–240.

Trape, J.-F., A. Tall, N. Diagne, O. Ndiath, A. B. Ly, J. Faye, F. Dieye-Ba, C. Roucher, C. Bouganali, A. Badiane, F. Diene Sarr, C. Mazenot, A. Touré-Baldé, D. Raoult, P. Druilhe, O. Mercereau-Puijalon, C. Rogier, and C. Sokhna. "Malaria Morbidity and Pyrethroid Resistance after the Introduction of Insecticide-treated Bed Nets Artemisinin-based Combination Therapies: A Longitudinal Study," *The Lancet Infectious Diseases*, vol. 11, no. 12 (2011), 925–932.

Trape, J.-F., A. Zoulani, and M. C. Quinet. "Assessment of the Incidence and Prevalence of Clinical Malaria in Semi-Immune Children Exposed to Intense Perennial Infections," *American Journal of Epidemiology*, vol. 126, no. 2 (1987), 193–201.

Tredre, R. F. *Malaria in the Forest Belt of the Gold Coast* (London: Ross Institute, London School of Hygiene and Tropical Medicine, n. d.).

Trigg, P. I., and A. V. Kondrachine. "Commentary: Malaria Control in the 1990s," *Bulletin of the World Health Organization*, vol. 76, no. 1 (1998), 11–16.

Turshen, M. *Privatizing Health Services in Africa* (New Brunswick, NJ: Rutgers University Press, 1999).

Ugwu, C. "Making-up Malaria Data: A Nigerian Example," IFRA-Nigeria Working Papers Series, no. 29. 31/05/2013. Available online: http://www.ifra-nigeria.org/IMG/pdf/making-up-malaria-data.pdf

United Nations Development Program. *Human Development Report 1991* (New York: Oxford University Press, 1991).

Utzinger, J., Y. Tozan, F. Doumani, and B. H. Singer. "The Economic Payoffs of Integrated Malaria Control in the Zambian Copperbelt between 1930 and 1950," *Tropical Medicine and International Health*, vol. 7, no. 8 (2002), 657–677.

Van den Berg, H. "Global Status of DDT and Its Alternatives for Use in Vector Control to Prevent Disease," *Environmental Health Perspectives*, vol. 117, no. 11 (2009), 1656–1663.

Van Nitsen, R. "Le paludisme chez l'enfant indigène," *Annales de la Société belge de médecine tropicale*, vol. 15 (1935), 229–268.

Vaucel, M. "Etat actuel du paludisme dans les colonies françaises," *Bullétin de la Société de pathologie exotique et de ses filiales*, vol. 39, nos. 1–2 (1946), 29–36.

Vercruysse, J., T. P. M. Schetters, D. P. Knox, P. Willadsen, and E. Claerebout, "Control of Parasitic Disease Using Vaccines: An Answer to Drug Resistance?,"

Revue scientifique et technique de l'Office International des Epizooties, vol. 26, no. 1 (2007), 105–115.

Verdrager, J. "Epidemiology of Emergence and Spread of Drug-Resistant Falciparum Malaria in Southeast Asia," *Southeast Asian Journal of Tropical Medicine and Public Health*, vol. 17, no. 1 (1986), 111–118.

Verhave, J. P. *The Moses of Malaria. Nicholaas H. Swellengrebel (1885–1970) Abroad and at Home* (Rotterdam: Erasmus Publishing, 2011).

Vialatte, C., and P. E. F. Sainte-Marie. "Autour du 'Mystère' de la fièvre quarte," *Bullétin de la Société de pathologie exotique et de ses filiales*, vol. 24 (1931), 280–285.

Vidal, L., A. Salam Fall, and D. Gadou. *Les professionnels de santé en Afrique de l'Ouest: Entre savoirs et pratiques: Paludisme, tuberculose et prévention au Sénégal et en Côte d'ivoire* (Paris: L'Harmattan, 2005).

Viegas de Ceita, J. G. "Malaria in São Tomé and Principe," in A. A. Buck (ed.), *Proceedings of the Conference on Malaria in Africa, Practical Considerations on Malaria Vaccines and Clinical Trials, Washington, DC, December 1–4, 1986* (Washington, DC: American Institute of Biological Sciences, 1987), 142–155.

Vincke, I. H. "Prophylaxie médicamenteuse de paludisme en zone rurale," *Bulletin of the World Health Organization*, vol. 11, nos. 4–5 (1954), 785–792.

Vincke I. H., P. G. Janssens, and J. Bafort. "Aspects de l'épidémiologie et de la lutte antipaludique en Afrique tropicale," *Bullétin de la Société de pathologie exotique*, vol. 59, no. 4 (1959), 483–492.

Waddington, C. J., and K. A. Enyimayew. "A Price to Pay: The Impact of User Charges in Ashanti-Akim District, Ghana," *International Journal of Health Planning and Management*, vol. 4, no. 1 (1989), 17–47.

Waddington, C., and K. A. Enyimayew. "A Price to Pay, Part 2: The Impact of User Charges in the Volta Region of Ghana," *International Journal of Health Planning and Management*, vol. 5, no. 4 (1990), 287–312.

Walker, K., and M. Lynch. "Contributions of *Anopheles* Larval Control to Malaria Suppression in Tropical Africa: Review of Achievements and Potential," *Medical and Veterinary Entomology*, vol. 21, no. 1 (2007), 2–21.

Walton, G. A. "On the Control of Malaria in Freetown, Sierra Leone. I. *Plasmodium falciparum* and *Anopheles gambiae* in Relation to Malaria Occurring in Infants," *Annals of Tropical Medicine and Parasitology*, vol. 41, nos. 3–4 (1947), 380–407.

Walton, G. A. "On the Control of Malaria in Freetown, Sierra Leone. II. Control Methods and the Effects upon the Transmission of *Plasmodium falciparum* Resulting from the Reduced Abundance of *Anopheles gambiae*," *Annals of Tropical Medicine and Parasitology*, vol. 413, no. 2 (1949), 117–139.

Warrell, D. A., and H M. Gilles (eds.). *Essential Malariology* (London: Arnold Publishers, 2002).

Watkins, W. M., and M. Mosobo. "Treatment of *Plasmodium falciparum* with Pyrimethamine-Sulfadoxine: Selective Pressure for Resistance Is a Function of Long Elimination Half-Life," *Transactions of the Royal Society of Tropical Medicine and Hygiene*, vol. 87, no. 1 (1993), 75–78.

Watson, M. "Malaria in Rhodesia and South Africa," *Journal of Tropical Medicine and Hygiene*, vol. 33, no. 23 (1 December 1930), 349–351.

Watson, M. "The Geographical Aspects of Malaria," *Geographical Journal*, vol. 49, no. 4 (1942), 161–172.

Watson, M. *African Highway: The Battle for Health in Central Africa* (London: John Murray, 1953).

Weatherall, R. "Malaria and the Opening Up of Central Africa," *Nature*, vol. 208, issue 5017 (1965), 1267–1269.

Webb, Jr., J. L. A. *Humanity's Burden: A Global History of Malaria* (New York: Cambridge University Press, 2009).

Webb, Jr., J. L. A. "The Long Shadow of Malaria Control in Tropical Africa," *The Lancet*, vol. 374 (5 December 2009), 1883–1884.

Webb, Jr., J. L. A. "The First Large-Scale Use of Synthetic Insecticides for Malaria Control in Tropical Africa," *Journal of the History of Medicine and Allied Sciences*, vol. 66, no. 3 (2011), 347–376.

Webb, Jr., J. L. A. "Malaria in Africa," *History Compass*, vol. 9, no. 3 (2011), 162–170.

Webb, Jr., J. L. A. "On Biomedicine, Transfers of Knowledge, and Malaria Treatments in Eastern North America and Tropical Africa," in D. M. Gordon and S. Krech III (eds.), *Indigenous Knowledge and the Environment in Africa and North America* (Athens: Ohio University Press, 2012), 53–68.

Webb, Jr., J. L. A. "Historical Epidemiology and Infectious Disease Processes in Africa," *Journal of African History*, vol. 54, no. 1 (2013), 3–10.

Webb, Jr., J. L. A. "Malaria Control and Eradication Projects in Tropical Africa, 1945–1965," in R. Bucala and F. Snowden (eds.), *The Global Challenge of Malaria: Past Lessons and Future Prospects* (New York: World Scientific Publishing, 2014), 35–56.

Weil, D. N. "Endemic Diseases and African Economic Growth: Challenges and Policy Responses," *Journal of African Economies*, vol. 19, AERC Suppl. 3 (2010), iii81-iii109.

Wilson, D. B. "Rural Hyper-Endemic Malaria in Tangayika Territory," *Transactions of the Royal Society of Tropical Medicine and Hygiene*, vol. 29, no. 6 (1936), 583–618.

Wilson, D. B. *Report of the Malaria Unit, Moshi, 1936* (Dar es Salaam: Government Printer, 1938).

Wilson, D. B. "Implications of Malarial Endemicity in East Africa," *Transactions of the Royal Society of Tropical Medicine and Hygiene*, vol. 32, no. 4 (1939), 435–465.

Wilson, D. B. *Report on the Control of Malaria in the Accra, Takoradi and Sekondi Areas* (Accra: Government Printing Office, 1946).

Wilson, D. B. "Malaria in the African," *Central African Journal of Medicine*, vol. 4, no. 2 (1958), 73–77.

Wilson, D. B. *Report on the Pare Taveta Scheme* (Dar es Salaam: Government Printer, 1960).

Wilson, D. B., P. C. C. Garnham, and N. H. Swellengrebel. "A Review of Hyperendemic Malaria," *Tropical Diseases Bulletin*, vol. 47, no. 8 (1947), 677–698.

Wilson, D. B., and M. E. Wilson. "The Manifestations and Measurement of Immunity to Malaria in Different Races," *Transactions of the Royal Society of Tropical Medicine and Hygiene*, vol. 30, no. 4 (1937), 431–448.

Wilson, D. B., and M. E. Wilson. "Control of *A. gambiae* on Coffee Estates," *East African Medical Journal*, vol. 16, no. 11 (1939–1940), 405–415.

Wilson, M. E., and D. B. Wilson. "Malarial Infectivity in African Soldiers in a Hyper-Endemic Area," *East African Medical Journal*, vol. 22 (1945), 295–297.

Winckel, C. W. F. "Comments on the Report of the Third Session of the Expert Committee on Malaria of the World Health Organization," *Documenta Neerlandica et Indonesica de Morbis Tropicis*, vol. 2, no. 3 (1950), 209–224.

World Health Organization. *Re-Examination of the Global Strategy of Malaria Eradication*, Official Record, No. 176, Annex 13 (Geneva: WHO, 1969).

World Health Organization. *Malaria Control in Countries Where Time-Limited Eradication Is Impracticable*, World Health Organization Technical Report Series no. 537 (Geneva: WHO, 1974).

Wone, I., and R. Michel. "Bilan de la chemioprophylaxie systématique par chloroquine au Sénégal, 1963–1966," *Médecine d'Afrique Noire*, no. 6 (June 1967), 267–269.

Zahar, A. R. "Vector Control Operations in the African Context," *Bulletin of the World Health Organization*, vol. 62, supplement (1984), 89–100.

Zulueta, J. de, G. W. Kafuko, J. R. Cullen, and C. K. Pedersen. "The Results of the First Year of a Malaria Eradication Project in Northern Kigezi," *East African Medical Journal*, vol. 38, no. 1 (1961), 1–26.

Zulueta, J. de, G. W. Kafuko, A. W. R. McCrae, J. R. Cullen, C. K. Pedersen, and D. F. B. Wasswa, "A Malaria Eradication Experiment in the Highlands of Kigezi (Uganda)," *East African Medical Journal*, vol. 41, no. 3 (1964), 102–120.

Index